CW00370269

Cardiac Nursing

Cardiac Nursing

Verity Wilson SRN RCNT DipN (Lond)
formerly Sister, Intensive Care Unit
St Bartholomew's Hospital, London
and Sister, Coronary Unit
The London Chest Hospital

Blackwell Scientific Publications

OXFORD LONDON
EDINBURGH BOSTON MELBOURNE

© 1983 by
Blackwell Scientific Publications
Editorial offices:
Osney Mead, Oxford OX2 0EL
8 John Street, London WC1N 2ES
9 Forrest Road, Edinburgh EH1 2QH
52 Beacon Street, Boston
    Massachusetts 02108, USA
99 Barry Street, Carlton
    Victoria 3053, Australia

Set by Typecast Photosetting, Kent
Printed and bound in Great Britain
by Billing and Sons Ltd, Worcester

DISTRIBUTORS

USA
    Blackwell Mosby Book Distributors
    11830 Westline Industrial Drive
    St Louis, Missouri 63141

Canada
    Blackwell Mosby Book Distributors
    120 Melford Drive, Scarborough
    Ontario, M1B 2X4

Australia
    Blackwell Scientific Book Distributors
    31 Advantage Road, Highett
    Victoria 3190

British Library
Cataloguing in Publication Data

Wilson, Verity
    Cardiac nursing.
    1.   Heart – Diseases
    2.   Cardiovascular disease nursing
    I.   Title
    616.1'2'0024613   RC681
    ISBN 0-632-00817-2

Contents

Preface

I have written this book for nurses and senior student nurses who want to understand the various causes and effects of cardiac disease processes while undertaking cardiac, cardiothoracic, or intensive care courses. It is also intended to encourage all nurses to use their knowledge and observation skills to assess and diagnose present and potential patient problems, then to intervene with appropriate nursing care.

I have arranged the chapters to begin with skills and techniques of assessment and investigation, followed by the anatomy and cardiovascular physiology of the normal heart. This is followed by a chapter on the normal electrocardiogram and how to read it, as well as arrhythmia diagnosis, appropriate intervention, and treatment by drugs or pacemakers. (This chapter could be used as reference only for some nurses or studied in depth by those working on a coronary care unit.) The causes, effects and treatment of heart failure are discussed in general, then the detailed nursing care required by patients in moderate heart failure, and the assessment of potential problems. This is followed by discussion of the nursing intervention and treatment for patients in severe failure and cardiogenic shock, including details of the intra-aortic balloon pump, cardiac arrest, and defibrillation procedures. Specific cardiac diseases are described including valve, congenital, and ischaemic disorders, together with their special investigation, treatment, and care. The last chapter deals with cardiac surgery including transplant surgery, the assessment of potential problems, and specific care from theatre through intensive care and recovery.

To increase ease of reading I have been unable to resist sexist terminology and have often referred to nurses (the majority of whom are female) as 'she', and patients (the majority of whom are male) as 'he'. I hope this will not offend male nurses or confuse nurses caring for female cardiac patients.

Verity Wilson, London 1983

Chapter 1
Introduction to cardiac patients and investigations

Cardiovascular disease takes the lives of more people than any other group of diseases, including neoplasms. Of the 580 000 deaths in England and Wales in 1980, half were due to cardiovascular disease. Most of the victims were over 55 years of age but the numbers of relatively young people who die are increasing every year. Some of these people will have died suddenly and unexpectedly, but many others suffer ill health of varying degrees for many years as a result of heart disease.

The incidence of rheumatic heart disease has, however, diminished due to improved standards of living, health care, and antibiotics. Nurses must therefore recognize the importance of their role in educating people to live healthier lives as more is learnt about the possible causes and means of reducing the risk of developing ischaemic and hypertensive heart disease. All nurses, both in the hospital and community, may be involved in the care of the cardiac patient and his family.

The patient may come under medical care from numerous sources: casualty, work, his own doctor, or following insurance examination or routine examination from baby clinics. Some patients may be in great physical distress, showing all or some of the features in Fig. 1.1. Many will appear physically asymptomatic on admission, but will be very worried and anxious. Much of the nursing time will be spent observing both the patient's overall well being, and the various measurements of cardiac performance and vascular response.

THE NURSING HISTORY

The nursing history considers the patient as a person who has individual and special facets to his personality. A forthcoming operation may cause great anxiety to one person, but relief to another. The nurse should try to understand the patient's individual pattern of life, anxieties and fears, and how to relieve or solve these fears. When these have been isolated and the information recorded, the nursing team should be more able to help that particular patient throughout the investigations, treatment, and return to as full a life as possible. From talking to the patient and observing him during routine admission procedures, the nurse can both allay the fears of the patient by giving information and reassurance and also gain much information about what the patient feels is the reason for his admission, what led up to the present illness, and how the patient is coping, both physically and mentally, with his cardiac problem. The nurse should encourage the patient to talk about his family, who is caring for those at home, who will be visiting and who, if anyone, will be able to assist the patient and his family during hospitalization and convalescence.

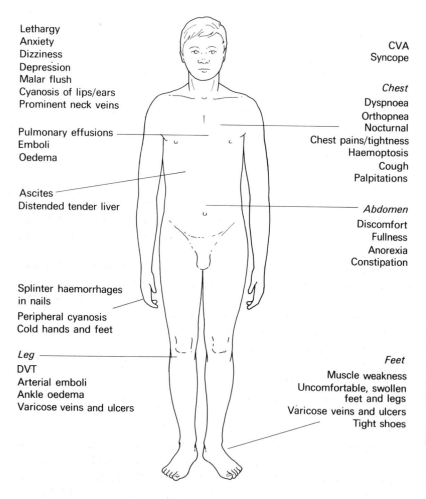

Fig. 1.1 Signs and symptoms of cardiac disease.

ASSESSING THE CARDIOVASCULAR STATE

Much of the nurse's contact with the patient occurs while she is measuring temperature, pulse, respiration and blood pressure. In addition to these, the skilled nurse should observe the patient's skin and general appearance, together with his mental and physical alertness, so as to build a picture of how effectively the heart is pumping and to what extent other body mechanisms are compensating for deficiencies in the cardiovascular system. The nurse should be continually thinking of what is happening physiologically and emotionally to the patient. Only then can she identify his needs.

Nurses observe the patient closely throughout the 24 hours; it is they who should notice any change in the patient's condition, and should therefore know what changes to look for, which are serious, and what action to take. The frequency of observations will depend on how rapidly changes are expected in the patient's progress, to monitor response to therapy and to detect any complications that could occur, e.g. infection hypotension, or heart failure.

The skin

Much useful information about the patient's condition can be gained by feeling the patient's skin as you talk to him or while carrying out nursing procedures. This is because changes in the peripheral blood flow, blood oxygen content and intestitial fluid volume are reflected in the skin and mucous membranes.

Note the skin colour and temperature, if it is dry or moist, and if oedema or dehydration are present. Skin under loose tension, e.g. at the back of the hand and at the neck, is commonly used to test for dehydration. If the patient is dehydrated, the skin will remain elevated in folds when it is gently pinched between the fingers.

If intestitial fluid is excessive, oedema will collect in dependent parts of the body: the feet and ankles will swell. However, if the patient is confined to bed then the sacrum, rather than the ankles, will show signs of oedema. To test for oedema, gently but firmly press your fingers into the swollen area, if the fingers leave indentations, pitting oedema is said to be present.

In congestive heart failure the veins in the hands and feet will appear full. The jugular venous pressure (JVP) will be elevated and can be measured, when the patient is lying in bed at a 45° angle, as centimeters above the clavicle (Fig. 1.2). In severe congestive failure, the JVP may be 5 – 10 cm elevated (*see* p. 11).

Another method of estimating the filling pressure of the right atrium is to raise the patient's hand and arm slowly until the veins empty. In health, this is usually at shoulder height. However, in dehydration, in a cold environment, or in poor cardiac output states, the hand veins may be collapsed even when they are lying at the patient's side.

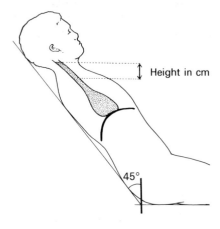

Height in cm

45°

Fig. 1.2   Measurement of jugular venous pressure (for details see text).

In normal health, at room temperature blood will be pumped to perfuse all tissues including the skin and mucous membranes which, if the haemoglobin (Hb) is normal and fully oxygenated, will appear pink. If more than 5 g of Hb per 100 ml of blood in the capillaries is uncombined with oxygen, the skin will have a bluish tinge called cyanosis. The cyanosis may be central or peripheral.

Central cyanosis is usually due to dangerously low intra-arterial levels of oxygen caused by a circulatory or respiratory malfunction — giving a bluish tinge to the skin over the chest and body. Peripheral cyanosis, however, occurs even if intra-arterial oxygen levels are adequate but peripheral capillary bloodflow is excessively slow, as seen in low cardiac output states where blood may be diverted to essential organs at the expense of the peripheries. The sluggish capillary flow to the hands and feet allows these tissues the time to extract more oxygen than usual from the Hb in their peripheral capillaries, hence the peripheries will appear blue.

More than 5 g of Hb may remain uncombined in persons with high Hb levels (polycythaemia) giving central cyanosis even if the blood is adequately oxygenated. Polycythaemia is a compensatory mechanism in some congenital heart and chronic respiratory conditions. Conversely, very anaemic persons will not appear cyanosed even with excessively low arterial oxygen levels.

Note if the fingernail beds are pink or bluish and compare with the colour of the lips and ears. Bruising or petechial haemorrhages, if present, could indicate coagulation disorders or emboli from the left heart.

A fall in blood pressure, hypoxia, pain, stress, or fear cause adrenaline release and stimulation of the vasomotor centre to bring about arteriolar vasoconstriction by increasing sympathetic tone. This response increases peripheral resistance to cause a rise in blood pressure (a compensatory mechanism); sweat glands are also stimulated causing the skin to become clammy. Skin temperature measurement is such an accurate guide that an electrical thermister on the foot is used in the shocked or the post cardiac surgery patient to indicate the level of tissue perfusion and cardiac output.

The nurse should compare signs detected from the skin with other signs, symptoms, and knowledge about the patient's diagnosis. Record and report any relevant observations.

Alertness

A dulled, vague or restless level of consciousness may be apparent to the nurse as she talks to the patient. A reduced blood or oxygen supply to the brain cells, as occurs in very low cardiac output states, cerebral emboli or hypoxia from lung disease could be the cause. The nurse should engage the patient in conversation to assess any change in mental state as she carries out other nursing procedures. Physical alertness and agility in movement when the patient walks or moves about in bed should be noted.

Lethargy is a complication of lowered cardiac output. Dizziness and loss of consciousness could occur suddenly with an inadequate cardiac output, due to arrhythmias, aortic stenosis or orthostatic hypotension. However, hypogylcaemia and cerebrovascular disease can also cause dizziness.

If changes have occurred, record other observations and immediately report any abrupt deterioration to the medical staff.

Temperature

Raised body temperature occurs as a response to infection, inflammation and raised metabolic rates, e.g. thyrotoxicosis. When cells are destroyed by infection, injury, or cancerous growth, neutrophil leucocytes release pyrogen which acts on the hypothalamus to raise the temperature. A raised body temperature acts both on the cardiac centre and also directly on the sinus node to increase the heart rate.

Inflammation from myocardial infarction, pulmonary embolism, or deep vein thrombosis will raise the temperature to about 38.5°C over 2–5 days, but inflammation does not usually cause rigors, night sweats or temperatures over 39°C. Accurate recording can greatly assist diagnosis, as different infections and inflammations have characteristic temperature charts. The nurse should identify those patients who may develop a temperature, and keep a 4 – 6 hourly chart on them so that early treatment can be given to prevent damage to the heart or other organs.

Heart rate

The heart rate should be counted at the apex to ensure accuracy. Peripheral pulses may be difficult to feel and count in patients with cardiovascular disease, especially if the patient has an arrhythmia or hypotension. However, the apex beat may be difficult to hear in obese patients. If a patient appears collapsed, feel for the carotid pulse which will be palpable if the heart is beating.

To plan how frequently it is necessary to record the heart rate, identify those patients in whom an altered heart rate may be significant to treatment. Patients with mitral valve disease and coronary disease may have a completely irregular rhythm called *atrial fibrillation* (AF). Some patients may have AF for many years and will tolerate this rhythm, but if a patient suddenly develops AF he may become hypotensive or shocked with acute heart failure.

Premature ectopic beats occur in normal hearts, especially after stimulation with caffeine or nicotine. Ectopics upset the normal heart rhythm and can be dangerous for patients with irritable hearts (post myocardial infarction for example), for those with electrolyte imbalance due to surgery or diuretic therapy, or for those taking digoxin.

Respiration

Respiration is an important and often badly recorded measurement. As well as the frequency counted over a whole minute, the nurse should note the depth and pattern of breathing, the chest movement, and whether accessory muscles are being used. Shortness of breath, or a change in breathing pattern, normally occurs on strenuous exertion, but the cardiac patient may become breathless on only mild exertion, before, during or after chest pain or palpitations, and associated with dizziness or anxiety. The nurse should observe and record these changes with other relevant information to aid diagnosis and treatment.

Blood pressure

Diagnosis and treatment rely heavily on accurate blood pressure recording and charting. The patient should be relaxed with his arm supported, the cuff should be a third of the width of the upper arm, and wrapped smoothly around the middle of the upper arm with the balloon over the artery. If the patient is receiving hypotensive therapy or is being investigated for orthostatic hypotension, his lying and standing pressures may be different, and therefore should be recorded separately.

Blood pressure = cardiac output × peripheral resistance

The systolic recording indicates the highest pressure generated by the left ventricle at systole (contraction). The diastolic pressure indicates the peripheral vascular resistance. The pressure can be altered by many variables: the vasomotor centre, arteriolar size, blood volume, drugs, and changing body demands.

The patient with hypertension may look deceptively fit, but may suffer headaches, blurred vision or breathlessness. If hypertension is left untreated the patient may suddenly develop heart failure, a stroke, ruptured aneurysm or other cardiovascular catastrophy.

Low blood pressure — hypotension — may result from a reduced cardiac output or reduced peripheral resistance. These two variables usually compensate each other, so if hypotension does occur it will be a late sign, and the patient will require urgent treatment to avoid irreparable damage to organs.

Pain or discomfort

Pains may occur in the chest for many reasons. The most common cardiac cause is from ischaemic heart disease, which alone accounts for more than half of all deaths due to cardiovascular disease. The lungs, airways, thoracic cage and great blood vessels may also produce pain in the chest, but so can other organs, e.g. the digestive system can produce severe pain in indigestion which may be mistaken for angina. Pain from heart disease may be referred to points distant from the heart, e.g. in the jaw, back, abdomen, or arms.

The patient may not complain of any pain, but the nurse may notice the patient's expression or a reluctance to move about in bed, which should prompt her to question the patient. The site of any pain, its character, whether dull or sharp, any precipitating factors, radiation, or relieving factors should be elicited, along with any other signs or symptoms such as breathlessness, palpitations, or dizziness. Record and report relevant information as appropriate.

DIFFERENTIAL DIAGNOSES OF CHEST PAIN

These are discussed in Table 4.1 (*see* p. 86); however, particular attention should be paid to the pain of angina.

Angina pain is the name given to the pain of coronary artery disease (*see* Chapter 7). The pain is typically dull, constricting and felt in the centre of the chest. It often radiates to the throat or left arm, and is precipitated by exercise or emotion. Rest or glyceryl trinitrate only relieve the pain but, if the pain lasts more than 20 minutes, myocardial infarction could be occurring. The patient may or may not be shocked. The pain typical of angina can occur in the presence of normal coronary arteries if oxygenated bloodflow through them is inadequate for other reasons. Patients with aortic stenosis commonly have angina, as do patients with hypertrophic obstructive cardiomyopathy (where the pain occurs when the patient lies down — angina decubitis).

SPECIAL CARDIAC INVESTIGATIONS

Cardiac catheterization and angiography

This investigation is carried out to reach a definite diagnosis or to conclusively rule out a particular condition, such as coronary artery disease. The test is invariably performed on all patients who may require cardiac surgery since other, less invasive, tests do not give the same wealth of information concerning the structure and function of the heart. The procedure will take place in a special theatre equipped with X-ray machinery.

Cardiac catheterization involves passing hollow radiopaque catheters via the brachial or femoral vein to investigate the right heart and through the brachial or femoral artery to reach the left heart, the coronary arteries, or the aorta. A cut down to the right brachial vessels, or a direct puncture to the femoral artery and/or vein, is performed under strict aseptic theatre technique and local anaesthesia.

Angiography involves the rapid injection of a radiopaque dye into the heart or blood vessels while the doctor operates and watches an image intensifier screen. Simultaneously a radiographer takes repeated X-ray films as directed by the doctor. The results obtained are:

1   Exact determination of cardiac output.
2   The detection, localization, and size of any intra- or extracardiac shunts by sampling blood oxygen in the cardiac chambers.
3   Measurement of the intracardiac and great vessel pressures.

4 Angiography shows the size and shape of the heart chambers and great vessels.

5 Cinecardiography takes films of the dye injection at 60 frames per second to record the movement of the heart structures as the dye is ejected from the heart. This not only shows defects of myocardial contraction, but also any valvular regurgitation.

6 Coronary angiography will pinpoint any stenoses or occlusions in the coronary arteries.

The procedure is rather unpleasant for the patient; the proximity of the X-ray machinery in the semi-darkness and the movement of the table to which the patient is strapped can promote extreme anxiety and discomfort. The patient should be kept informed of the proceedings in a manner that will help reduce anxiety, and should be warned to expect a sudden burning or bursting sensation when dye is injected into the heart.

A general anaesthetic is not given, except to young children, since it would prevent the patient telling the doctor that he was experiencing chest pain or breathlessness. Also a general anaesthetic alters blood oxygenation and cardiac output and could result in misleading information.

Catheterization and angiography have a mortality and morbidity rate, and are especially risky for the seriously ill infant. Complications may be transient or major and include ventricular tachycardia or fibrillation, perforation of the heart or great vessels, and emboli to the brain, lungs, or major vessels. The brachial or femoral artery used for the procedure may become occluded by spasm or thrombosis formation but this should respond to heparinization. If it does not, embolectomy and arterial repair will be necessary. A reaction to the dye used can occur, varying from a rash to laryngeal spasm and anaphylaxis.

NURSING CARE

Some of the preceding problems can be guarded against. The patient will have the procedure explained to him by a doctor before signing a consent form. He is prepared as for theatre and fasted to reduce the risk of inhaling vomit should cardiac arrest occur. The site over the right brachial artery should be shaved and washed to reduce any infection risk. A narcotic or sedative premedication helps to allay anxiety and pain and so reduces catecholamine release which can aggrevate the arrhythmia risk. An informed and constantly present nurse can greatly reassure the patient. Full resuscitation equipment should always be ready for use.

Following the procedure, a pressure dressing will be applied to the wound and, on return to the ward, the artery and vein used should be kept in view in case of haemorrhage. The limb should be kept straight to prevent turbulence of bloodflow at the incision with subsequent thrombus formation. If the femoral approach has been used the patient will usually stay in bed for 12 – 18 hours to prevent flexing the hip more than 40°. The limb should be inspected for pulse, colour, warmth, and sensation; any deterioration in perfusion should be notified immediately.

If a reaction to the dye occurs it is usually immediate and hydrocortisone and antihistamine will be given in the angiography department. However, a reaction may be delayed until the patient is back in the ward, so the patient should be closely observed. Pulse, respiration, and blood pressure as well as limb perfusion checks as previously explained should be recorded frequently for 4 – 6 hours.

Echocardiography

This is a non-invasive and totally safe investigation which can be carried out by an experienced doctor or technician at the bedside. A machine passes sounds through the patient's chest and records the echoes heard when the sound is reflected from intracardiac structures. The echoes are displayed on a screen and a printout can clearly show pericardial effusions, the thickness of the ventricular septum and walls, and the movement of the heart valves, especially the mitral valve. Also vegetations on the heart valves may be clearly seen.

NURSING CARE

Nursing care will involve privacy, explanation and positioning the patient comfortably on a few pillows. The operator will place a small microphone or recording piece over the patient's skin, using a little ultrasound gel.

Nuclear angiography or thalium scan

This procedure uses intravenous radioisotopes that migrate to active heart muscle. When the patient is scanned, only muscle that is alive with a good coronary blood supply will show up. Ischaemic areas, either at rest or after exercise can be revealed, as well as infarcted areas. This test may be used before angiography as it has fewer complications and may in some patients eliminate the need to proceed to angiography.

Cardiac biopsy

This procedure will be carried out in the angiography department on patients with suspected cardiomyopathy or for those following heart transplantation who are suspected of rejecting. The care and procedure are similar to cardiac catheterization.

Electrophysiological studies (His bundle electrocardiogram)

Patients with recurrent tachycardia who are resistant to drug therapy may have accessory pathways within the atrium and bundle of His that can be divided by cryosurgery once they have been isolated. This investigation studies the passage of normal and paced impulses from the sinus node and atria, through the AV node and bundle of His. Abnormal pathways, if present, may be identified.

The procedure is similar to cardiac catheterization, using pacing and recording electrodes passed via a vein into the right atrium and ventricle. Pre- and post-investigation care will be similar to that involved in catheterization with particular awareness of any arrhythmias.

Exercise ECG

This is carried out on patients with an inconclusive history of angina but who have a normal ECG. A resting ECG will be recorded, then the patient will be exercised, by pedalling an exercise bicycle or running on a treadmill while the ECG rhythm is observed. ECG s are recorded at two-minute intervals for six minutes, or until any changes return to the resting ECG. T wave inversion, ST segment depression, bundle branch blocks, axis change, or arrhythmias may develop.

A doctor should always be present throughout the test and, if the patient experiences pain, the exercise should be stopped immediately. Glyceryl trinitrate and full rescusitation equipment should be readily available.

CVP AND MONITORING PROCEDURES

The central venous pressure

Central venous pressure (CVP) is caused by the blood returning from the great veins in the thorax to the right atrium, and is the filling pressure or preload of the right heart. It indicates the heart's ability to accommodate the venous return.

In cardiogenic shock and congestive heart failure, the CVP will be raised because the heart is unable to pump all the blood it receives from the veins into the arteries. Back pressure of blood will build up in the heart chambers and large veins. A low CVP indicates that there is not enough blood returning to the heart, due to haemorrhage, excessive diuresis, sweating, or inappropriate vasodilation. CVP is measured via an intravascular catheter.

INTRAVASCULAR CATHETERIZATION

Insertion
Aseptically, and using local anaesthetic, a cannula is passed by percutaneous puncture into a large vein. The antecubital, the subclavian, or most commonly the internal jugular vein is used. The cannula is attached to a manometer tubing and giving set which contains an isotonic solution, usually 5% dextrose. To check that the cannula is within a great vein in the thorax, watch the fluid in the manometer: it should swing as the pressures within the thorax change with respiration.

Precautions
Pain and anxiety. Local anaesthetic of 1% lignocaine should be used at the insertion site. The patient will be tipped head down for probably 10 – 15 minutes and his face may be covered in green towels. The nurse and doctor should explain in simple terms before the procedure begins what they are doing and why. A sedative such as intravenous diazepam may need to be given for the patient who is in shock, restless or confused. Patients who are also dyspnoeic require continual reassurance from the nurse.

Air embolism. If the subclavian or internal jugular approach is used, the patient should be lying in a head down position. This helps to fill the veins making it easier for the doctor to insert the cannula, and reduces the risk of air entering the cannula and hence the vein as the manometer line is connected.

Sepsis. A full aseptic technique should be used, with dressing pack, iodine for skin preparation, gloves and face mask. Afterwards the site can be sprayed with povidone iodine, then securely covered with a clear adhesive dressing. This facilitates observation of the insertion site for inflammation or haematoma and should be changed only when necessary — about every three days. If a dry dauze dressing and strapping are used, the dressing will need to be removed and inspected daily. Care is needed not to dislodge the cannula during re-dressing and the doctor may suture the line in position.

Trauma. A pneumothorax or haemothorax can be caused if a blood vessel or lung is punctured. A hydrothorax could occur if the cannula is not within the vein, allowing the infusion fluid to fill the thorax. The doctor will check that he has entered a vein by the free flowing back of blood into the infusion set when the infusion bag is held near the floor for a second or two. A chest X-ray should be taken after insertion to check that the catheter tip is correctly positioned as well as for pneumothorax.

CVP INTERPRETATION

CVP is measured with the patient on his back, in the position in which he is nursed. The level of the right atrium may be taken as the anterior or mid-axillary line, if the patient is nursed head up, or at the sternal notch if the patient is lying flat.

After levelling the zero on the manometer to the right atrium according to hospital procedure, the tap at the manometer is turned to fill the column from the infusion. When this has been done, the infusion is stopped and the column to the patient is opened. The column will fall to a level which you should note in cm of water. In health, the reading should be about 5 – 10 cm. If it is higher than 15 cm, suspect cardiac failure, overinfusion, tamponade, pulmonary oedema, or pulmonary embolism. If it is between zero and —10 cm, suspect hypovolaemia.

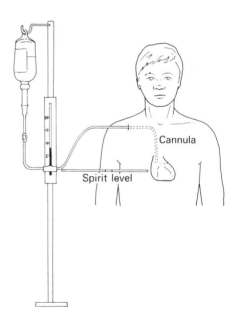

Fig. 1.3 Positioning of the CVP manometer.

Swan–Ganz catheter

Left ventricular preload is left atrial pressure. This can be directly measured with a catheter inserted during open heart surgery. To measure left atrial pressure indirectly, a Swan–Ganz catheter (Fig. 1.4.) is passed via a vein through the right heart and into the pulmonary artery (PA). This catheter is placed using similar aseptic techniques as for a CVP line or pacing wire; however, in order to direct the catheter through the heart, it has a small balloon on its end. This balloon is inflated so the flow of blood travelling through the heart carries the catheter into a small pulmonary artery where it wedges. This is as near to the left atrium as it is possible to get. The pressure sensor at the catheter tip reflects the pressure ahead of it, i.e. the left atrial pressure or pulmonary artery capillary wedge pressure (PACWP).

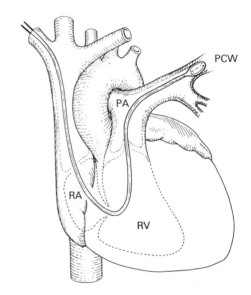

Fig. 1.4 A Swan–Ganz catheter wedged in the pulmonary artery. RA= right atrium, RV = right ventricle, PA = pulmonary artery, PCW = pulmonary capillary wedge.

PRECAUTIONS

In addition to the precautions discussed above for CVP measurement, the following should be noted.

Arrhythmias
These occur during insertion and removal as the catheter passes through the heart. Watch the monitor for ectopics and tachycardias. Remove the catheter slowly to prevent the tip flicking and irritating the endocardium.

Pulmonary embolism. When the catheter has been inserted and the wedge pressure recorded (Fig 1.5), the balloon is allowed to deflate so that the catheter falls back into the pulmonary artery. The monitor will show a pulmonary artery trace. If the balloon remains inflated or the catheter remains wedged, the lung served by that artery will not receive blood and will die as if a pulmonary embolism had occurred. The tracing should be observed frequently for this complication and, if it is suspected, the doctor should be notified immediately: he will withdraw the catheter slightly.

WEDGE PRESSURE RECORDING

The nurse may be asked to record hourly wedge pressures. This is done by slowly introducing one ml of air or CO_2 into the balloon while watching the monitor tracing. When the catheter wedges (*see* Fig. 1.5) the mean pressure or end diastolic pressure is recorded. The syringe is removed from the balloon line and the tracing should revert to the larger pulmonary artery trace. If you are unable to wedge the line, call the technician or doctor; do not add more and more air as the balloon may have burst.

Transfusion of plasma, or regulation of vasodilators and inotropic infusions may be requested according to the wedge pressure: in normal health 2 – 10 mmHg would be acceptable, but 10 – 18 mmHg may be ideal for a failing heart that requires high filling pressures. Remember that the pressure will be higher if the patient is ventilated, and even higher if positive end expiratory pressure is added. A very raised pressure would overfill and strain the left atrium and ventricle to increase failure and pulmonary oedema. A low filling pressure will produce a smaller stroke volume so that a tachycardia will occur to maintain cardiac output.

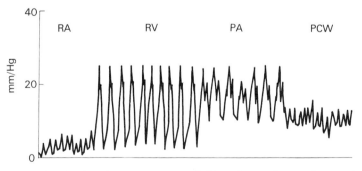

Fig. 1.5   The changing pressures recorded by a Swan–Ganz catheter as it is advanced into the wedge position.

Arterial monitoring

An arterial line is the most accurate method of observing changes in the blood pressure, and is used for a period of one or more days in critically ill patients. It has the additional advantage that repeated samples for blood estimations can be taken from this line.

INSERTION

Under local anaesthetic a disposable cannula is inserted aseptically by an anaesthetist — commonly into the radial artery. The cannula is attached by a fluid-filled polythene manometer line to a transducer which converts the pressure changes into a wave form that can be viewed continually on an oscilloscope. The fluid used is heparinized Hartmann's or normal saline, and is delivered under pressure through a continual low volume flushing device — an intraflow — which delivers 3 ml/hour.

COMPLICATIONS

Concealed haemorrhage. If the arterial line becomes disconnected, a large volume of blood could be lost. The limb with the line in should always be exposed to detect haemorrhage. Secure but non-occlusive strapping should be used, splinting is not usually necessary or effective.

Air emboli. Any air in the manometer line entering the arterial line would travel to the tissues served by that artery, e.g. a necrotic finger could result from even a very small air bubble in a radial line. If drugs were inadvertently given into the arterial line, instead of a venous line, serious tissue damage would result.

Ischaemia. This may occur if the artery is occluded by the cannula. The perfusion of the limb extremities can be tested by comparing the colour, temperature, and capillary perfusion with the other limb.

Aneursym formation. A weakness in the artery wall may develop due to prolonged use of an arterial cannula. The nurse should observe the site of insertion for any inflammation, haematoma or swelling. When the cannula is removed, firm direct finger pressure must be applied for at least five minutes, followed by a dry pressure dressing.

Fluid calculations. In babies and small children, the amount of fluid used to flush the line, and the quantity of blood taken as samples or spilt by disconnection must be included in the fluid chart.

To record a 12 lead ECG

An ECG is often one of the first tests the patient will have on admission to casualty, coronary care unit, or on the ward urgently after any abrupt change in his condition. The nurse can help to allay anxiety by explaining to the patient that the test is quite painless, that it is frequently carried out on patients with chest pain, breathlessness, or palpitation (whichever is appropriate to the particular patient), and that, though a simple test, it can give valuable information concerning the heart.

The bed should be screened to give privacy and to allow the patient to relax. Relaxation is important as muscle tremor or sweating can produce a technically poor ECG which will be more difficult to interpret.

The patient should be resting comfortably on pillows with head and limbs supported. The lower legs and arms should be exposed, the bed clothes can be turned up at the foot of the bed. The chest need not be exposed until necessary. Women with large breasts may need to be placed a little flatter in bed so that the chest electrode can be correctly positioned.

PREPARATION

A little electrode gel is applied with a spatula or a saline-impregnated disposable pad to the flat area of each lower leg and arm. A flat area is chosen so that the whole of the electrode plate will be in contact with the skin when it is firmly but not tightly applied with a rubber strap.

The cables are attached to the electrode plates, great care being taken to attach the appropriate cable to the correct limb. The cables are usually labelled or colour coded with the colour key painted on the individual machine. The cables should be free of tangles, should not drag or pull on the patient, and the operator should not touch the bed or the cable so that interference does not occur.

THE MACHINE

There are various components of the machine with which the nurse should familiarize herself: the stylus, the paper, calibration and sensitivity, and lead selector.

Stylus

The stylus either burns the electrical wave forms onto wax paper or it draws them with ink. If the tracing produced is too faint or too dark the stylus heat should be adjusted. Ink machines should constantly adjust their ink flow but may need priming, the ink bottle may have to be changed, or the stylus may be blocked and require careful cleaning or replacement. The stylus pressure on the paper can also be adjusted. If the machine is handled roughly, especially during paper changing, or the lead selector is left on between leads, then the stylus can become bent and damaged. Before recording from any lead, allow the stylus to return to a central and stable position. Adjust the position of the stylus as necessary before running the paper.

Paper

The paper will be 4 or 5 cm wide and pulled at a speed of 25 mm per second. The squares on the paper therefore represent time. Most machines have the facility to double the speed to 50 mm per second to allow closer scrutiny of abnormalities. Changing the paper is usually easier than it looks although care must be taken not to damage the stylus. Read the manufacturer's instructions and use the correct paper for the individual machine.

Calibration and sensitivity

Calibration is necessary to standardize the height of the QRS complexes so that comparison with previous and future ECG recordings can be made. ECG recordings are usually taken at a standard sensitivity so that a 1 mV signal input gives a deflection of 1 cm on the paper. Most machines also have settings to halve or double the sensitivity — and hence the QRS size — i.e. 2.0 mV per cm and 0.5 mV per cm.

Before a recording is made the accuracy of the 1 mV per cm setting is tested and a record is made of the calibration at the beginning of each tracing; this is mounted with the record from the 12 leads. This test is performed with the lead selector turned to the 'standardize position' when a 1 mV signal from the calibrate button is recorded with the paper running. The tracing should be clean and sharply defined: if it is not, ensure that the recording stylus is clean. The upward deflection should be 1 cm in amplitude (10 small squares on the graph paper), with an initial overshoot of 5%: if it is not, adjust the sensitivity control, stylus pressure, or damping control as necessary. The 5% overshoot is considered the optimum required to achieve high frequency response.

The 2 mV setting is used to record high voltage signals (greater than 4 or 5 mV) which are commonly found in the V leads, particularly with children. The change in sensitivity should be recorded on the paper and written, for example, as $V_3\frac{1}{2}$.

The lead selector and recording

When the patient has been connected to the machine and the sensitivity checked and recorded with the patient's name and date, the selector is switched in turn to each lead; the bipolar leads I, II and III then the unipolar leads AVR, AVL, and AVF. A check to ensure that the leads and cables are correctly attached to the patient should be made if lead I is negative or AVR positive to be sure the leads are not reversed.

Record four or five complexes on each lead, and label the tracing before moving on to the next lead. After each change in lead selected allow the base line to settle and observe the stylus flicking with each QRS complex before running the paper. In this manner a neat recording will be obtained which will be easier to interpret.

To record the chest leads attach the chest electrode to the patient cable. Explain what you are doing to the patient, expose the chest and apply a little paste before applying the chest electrode, which is usually of the suction type. Fig. 3.21, (p. 53) shows the positions in which to place the chest electrodes. It is most important for interpretation and comparison that the correct positions are used. Turn the lead selector to V to record each lead but, between changes in electrode position, turn the lead selector to a neutral position to protect the stylus. While recording the chest leads it is still necessary to have the limb leads attached.

When the recording is complete, remove the electrodes and wipe dry any gel from the patient's skin with a tissue, rearrange the bedclothes and make the patient comfortable. Wash the electrodes and straps in soap and water and store the machine ready for re-use. The ECG should now be mounted on paper or card, according to the hospital procedure. Clearly label each lead, and remember to include the 1 mV standardization.

ARTEFACTS (*see also* p. 20)

Somatic tremor

An irregular fine variation is superimposed on the baseline and is caused by electropotentials from active muscle. This results from a nervous patient who is not relaxed or whose limbs are not properly supported on the bed. To avoid this the patient should be warm, relaxed and reassured. Even moving the head to watch the operator or talking will cause somatic tremor. In elderly patients or those with Parkinson's disease it may be impossible to obtain a perfect reading.

Mains interference

Mains interference produces a saw-tooth type of artefact on the tracing which will blur the recording. It may be due to interference from nearby equipment or increased mains wiring in the walls. Any unnecessary equipment, e.g. electrical thermometers, should be turned off while the recording is made but take care when turning off equipment in an intensive or coronary care unit! The plug should be an earthed, 3 pin plug and the wires must not be broken or the plug or socket faulty. A common and easily corrected cause is inadequate patient-to-lead contact. Check the electrodes and their connections and also make sure that neither the patient nor the operator is touching the metal of the bed. Other electrical hazards are mentioned on p. 21.

Baseline drift
This may spoil an otherwise clear recording, and may be due to the patient breathing heavily or the cable being too taut. Observe the stylus for a few seconds before running the paper to allow the baseline to settle and the machine to stabilize. This drift or break in recording may be more marked while recording the chest leads, especially in women with large breasts. The patient could be asked to breathe quietly just at the time the paper is running.

Monitoring

In many ways the procedure of ECG recording is similar to that of monitoring a patient. Monitoring affords observation without the need of repeatedly disturbing the patient to feel his pulse. Its purpose is to obtain a clear, continuous tracing over several days without causing any anxiety or discomfort to the patient and with the fewest possible electrical hazards. Before the electrodes are applied the patient should be lying comfortably in bed and should be screened. However, once everything is connected, this should not prevent the patient from moving freely about in bed and, should a wire become disconnected, a nurse can easily reconnect it.

EQUIPMENT AND TECHNIQUE

A mains or battery cardiac monitor, patient cable, electrode leads and pre-gelled silver chloride electrodes. Possibly soap, water, razor, towel and dry gauze will be required. Preparation is as described on p. 17.

The lead most commonly used is a modified Lead V_1, as this clearly shows arrhythmias, conduction abnormalities, and from which ventricle ectopic beats (if any) are occurring. To modify the lead, place the positive lead over the 4th intercostal space anteriorly, the negative lead near the left shoulder, and the indifferent lead near the right clavicle (Fig. 1.6).

INTERFERENCE

AC interference may produce a saw-tooth type of artefact. If the electrodes have been attached for many days the gel may be dry, resulting in poor patient contact. The electrodes, cables, and nearby equipment should be checked. To maintain a clear tracing and continuous monitoring even when the patient moves about, the cable and electrode wires should not be allowed to tangle, drag, or pull. Looping the wire and clipping it to the night or bed clothes may prevent this.

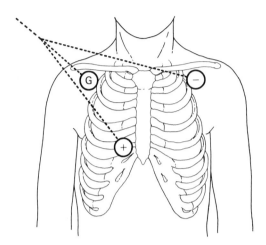

Fig. 1.6   Position of the monitor electrodes for a modified lead V1.

ELECTRICAL HAZARDS

All electrical equipment should be regularly checked and maintained by the medical electronics department or the manufacturers. Equipment that is suspected of being faulty, for example frayed cable, should be removed from use and clearly labelled. To prevent damage to equipment, staff or patients, ensure that the cable will not become trapped in back rests, that cable lengths are not longer than necessary to minimize current leak, and that water (or spilt intravenous fluid) is not able to get into electrical points.

If the patient has a transvenous pacing wire, Swan–Ganz catheter or long intravenous line, even a small current leak contacting these lines could be transmitted via the fluid column or pacing wire directly to the myocardium, causing ventricular fibrillation.

Chapter 2
The normal heart

The heart can be thought of as two muscular pumps. The right heart receives blood from the venae cavae and pumps blood under low pressure through the pulmonary circulation. The left heart receives oxygenated blood from the lungs and pumps blood under high pressure through the muscular and elastic arteries to all body tissues and organs in varying amounts depending on tissue needs.

Early in embryonic life the heart forms from a fold in a blood vessel (*see* Fig. 6.1). The structure of the heart is very like that of an artery in that it has three layers, an endocardial layer of squamous epithelium that lines all intracardiac structures, a thick muscular myocardial layer, and a surrounding fibrous pericardium (Fig. 2.1).

The lungs offer little vascular resistance compared to the systemic peripheral vessels, hence the left heart walls are thicker than the right because of the much greater work necessary to pump blood through the systemic circulation. The heart muscle is supplied with blood by the coronary arteries which arise behind the aortic valve cusps (see Chapter 7).

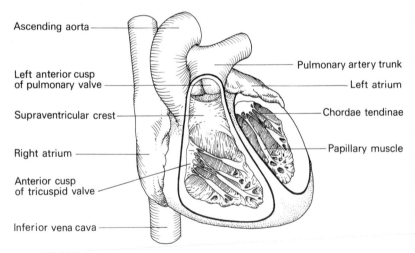

Ascending aorta

Left anterior cusp of pulmonary valve

Supraventricular crest

Right atrium

Anterior cusp of tricuspid valve

Inferior vena cava

Pulmonary artery trunk

Left atrium

Chordae tendinae

Papillary muscle

Fig. 2.1 Interior of the heart.

The valves (Fig. 2.2)

The direction of bloodflow within the heart is maintained by four valves made of fibrous tissue which sit in a fibrous ring called the *annulus*. The two atrioventricular valves are like parachutes tethered to the ventricles by chordae tendineae and papillary muscles, the pulmonary and aortic valves have semi-lunar cusps.

If these valves become damaged by rheumatic fever or by bacterial endocarditis, scarring can occur which will cause the valves to narrow (stenosis). Blood will be unable to pass through the valves freely, so the preceding muscular chamber will become engorged with blood and stressed. Similar effects occur if the valves become misshapen by disease and do not close properly, thus causing blood to flow back (regurgitate) into the chamber it has just left, e.g. mitral valve regurgitation causes the pressure in the left atrium to rise, in turn raising the pressure in the pulmonary veins. Disturbance to respiration and gaseous exchange may then occur, eventually leading to life-threatening pulmonary oedema.

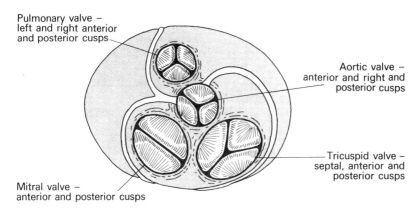

Pulmonary valve – left and right anterior and posterior cusps

Aortic valve – anterior and right and posterior cusps

Tricuspid valve – septal, anterior and posterior cusps

Mitral valve – anterior and posterior cusps

Fig. 2.2 The heart valves from above.

The endocardium

The endocardial lining covers all intracardiac structures and is smooth squamous epithelium. If roughened by disease, thrombi may cling to the surface giving rise to emboli that may dislodge and inflict damage to brain, kidneys, or limbs.

The myocardium

The cardiac muscle is unique in that it contracts and relaxes spontaneously throughout life. Its arrangement of muscle fibres into a latticework around the conical-shaped ventricles causes the blood to be squeezed, by coordinated contraction, into the arteries. The network of fibres can stretch and contract to accommodate and discharge an ever-changing venous return.

The muscle fibres are striated, have definite nuclei, and are divided by intercalated discs. The fibres are composed of two types of interlocking filaments, actin and myocin; when stimulated to contract, these slide over each other to shorten and thicken the muscle mass. Because the fibres divide and connect with each other in a latticework arrangement, the muscle is described as a *syncytium mass*. This means that if one part of the muscle mass is stimulated, the impulse will pass throughout the muscle fibres causing them all to shorten, so causing a coordinated cardiac contraction. The heart is composed of two separate syncytium masses, the atria and ventricles, if one part of a ventricle is stimulated the impulse will spread to both ventricles but not usually to the atria. If one atrium is stimulated, an impulse will be passed to the other atrium, causing them both to contract. The impulse can only be passed from the atria to the ventricles via the communicating atrioventricular node, then on to the ventricular muscle mass using the heart's own conducting system as described on p. 25.

If the muscle fibres are damaged by inflammatory disease, become deprived of oxygen from coronary artery disease, or are overstretched from hypertension or valve disease, the pumping efficiency of the heart will be impaired. The heart will no longer be able to adapt to changes in venous return or increase cardiac output during times of need. Heart failure will follow.

The pericardium

Overdistension of the heart is limited by the fibrous pericardial sac in which the heart sits. The pericardium has two layers, much like the pleura. On relaxation and contraction of the heart, friction between the two surfaces is eliminated by the small amount of serous fluid between them. If this lubrication is lost due to inflammation, the patient will experience chest pain and a pericardial friction rub will be heard by stethoscope. Should fibrosis follow inflammation, or the pericardium become filled with fluid or blood, the filling capacity of the heart will be restricted, so inhibiting the venous return entering the heart and lowering cardiac output.

The conducting system (Fig. 2.3)

The stimulus for the heart to contract is brought about by its own conducting system. All heart tissue has the ability to initiate impulses, to conduct these impulses to other cardiac cells, and to contract. Certain areas, however, are specialized.

The sinus node is a group of cells in the right atrium, lying at the junction of the right atrial appendage and the superior vena cava and acting as the pacemaker of the heart. The nodes are a collection of fibres covered in a perinodal capsule.

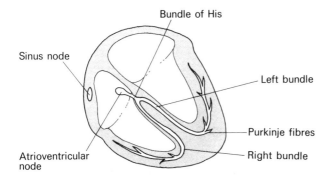

Fig. 2.3   Conducting tissue of the heart.

DEPOLARIZATION

The sinus node spontaneously and rhythmically discharges electrical impulses which are then conducted via special fibres through both atria to the atrioventricular node. This node lies between the coronary sinus and the tricuspid valve ring. The impulse is slowed by the AV node to allow the atria time to respond to the electrical impulse, i.e. to contract to push blood into the ventricles. The impulse is then passed by the bundle of His, left posterior, left anterior and right bundle branches and eventually the Purkinje fibres pass the impulse to all ventricular muscle causing ventricular activation and contraction.

This period of electrical activity is called *depolarization*, the mechanical activity of contraction is called *systole*. Following depolarization the heart muscle is termed *refractory* in that it cannot now pass impulses, or contract in response to impulses, until a period of adjustment of electrolytes by the cell membranes has occurred; this adjustment is called *repolarization*.

These electrical events take less than 0.4 seconds to occur. Mechanical systole occurs just after the electrical impulse, and there is then a period of muscle relaxation to allow the heart to fill with blood from the veins. This resting state is called *diastole*. The whole cycle from systole to the end of diastole takes about 0.8 seconds if the heart is beating 75 times a minute.

RESTING MEMBRANE POTENTIAL

The electrical events of depolarization and repolarization are not really an electrical phenomenon in the same sense as electrons flowing through conductors in an electric circuit, rather it is chemical in nature and involves the movement of ions (either positvely or negatively charged atoms) back and forth across cell membranes. The cell membranes can permit the movement of large quantities of positively charged sodium ions (Na^+) and it is the rapid shift of sodium in or out of the cell that mediates the electrical activity. In health there is six times more potassium than sodium within the cell, the sodium is actively removed from the cell by a sodium 'pump', so creating an electrical difference across the cell membrane. In this resting state of the cell, the potential voltage across the membrane is –90 millivolts (mV).

ACTION POTENTIAL

Should the cell be stimulated by an electric current, or an overwhelming flow of sodium ions enter the cell, an electric current will flow to other cells in a chain reaction of depolarization. The action potential will have been reached.

DEPOLARIZATION ACTION POTENTIAL   (Fig. 2.4)

Stage 0 The resting polarized cell is electrically stimulated and the cell membrane becomes permeable to sodium (Na^+); this then passes into the cell to cause rapid depolarization and movement of potassium (K^+) out of the cell. Thus the inside of the cell becomes positively charged in relation to the outside of the cell and contraction occurs.
Stage 1 A period of rapid repolarization occurs as sodium ions are pumped out via the cell membrane.
Stage 2 Gradual repolarization follows – this is called the *plateau* phase. Sodium ions are removed, and potassium ions and calcium enter the cell.
Stage 3 This is the final rapid phase of repolarization.
Stage 4 The cell reverts to a resting polarized state, with a resting potential of –90 mV.

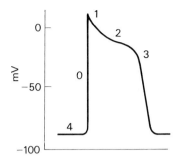

Fig. 2.4 Action potential of contractile and pacemaker cell.

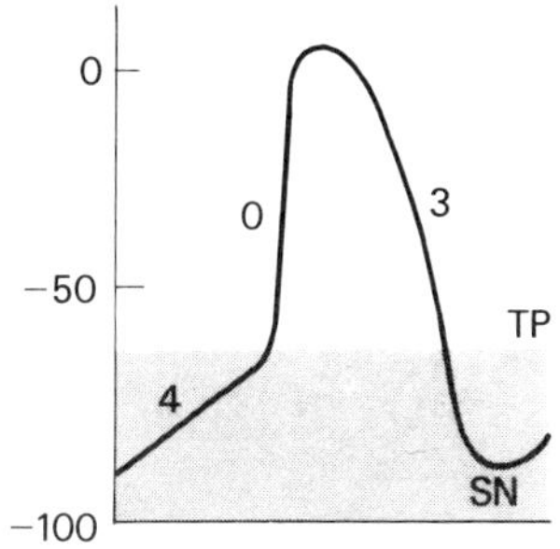

Fig. 2.5 Spontaneous depolarization of pacemaker cell (for details see text). TP = threshold potential, SN = supernormal phase.

THE SPONTANEOUS DEPOLARIZATION OF PACEMAKER CELLS

Pacemaking cells differ in all phases, most especially in phase 4 where slow diastolic depolarization automatically occurs in a regular manner until the threshold for spontaneous depolarization is reached. This drift to threshold is most marked in the sinus node, which automatically and regularly depolarizes at 80 – 100 times per minute. It is also the quickest heart tissue to repolarize and has the following cycle:

Phase 0 More gradual depolarization.

Phase 1 No overshoot to positive as for non-pacemaking muscle cell.

Phase 2 and 3 Quicker repolarization without plateau.

Phase 4 Spontaneous leak of sodium into the cell, until the threshold potential is reached. Spontaneous depolarization occurs.

Should the sinus node fail to discharge or the impulse be blocked, the atrioventricular node (as the next fastest depolarizing pacemaking cell) will initiate an impulse to produce an escape beat or rhythm. Following myocardial infarction, electrolyte imbalance, hypoxia or cardiac surgery, the threshhold potential is lowered in the affected cells. Automatic premature depolarization may occur to give ectopic beats. Should these ectopic beats occur while normal cells are at phases 2 and 3, i.e. repolarization (the T wave on the ECG) when the cell membrane is unstable, ventricular tachycardia or fibrillation can occur. This is therefore called the *vulnerable* period of the cardiac cycle.

Myocardial infarction and certain drugs extend repolarization, i.e. the QT interval on the ECG, and the patient may be more susceptible to ventricular fibrillation with this extension of the vulnerable period.

Heart sounds

The valves open and close due to the changing pressures within the heart chambers and arteries during the cardiac cycle (Figs. 2.6 and 2.7). The mechanical event of systole can be felt at the pulse or heard at the apex of the heart with a stethoscope. The sounds heard are from the two types of

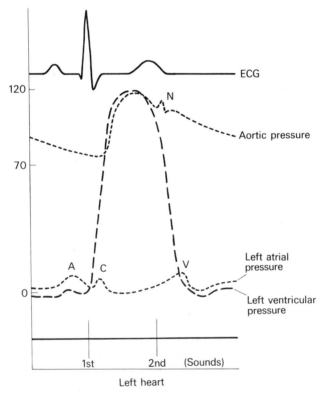

Fig 2.6   The cardiac cycle showing pressures in the aorta, left ventricle and left atrium.   A = atrial contraction, C = aortic valve opens, AV valves close, V = AV valve opens, N = dicrotic notch, aortic valve closes.

valves snapping shut at the beginning and end of systole. The first sound is of the mitral and tricuspid valves closing, the second sound is of the aortic and pulmonary valves closing.

The left and right heart valves close simultaneously in health, the left heart valves contributing most to the sound heard; however, should the valves close asyncronously, the right and left valve closure sounds will be split. This splitting of the heart sounds is important in diagnosis.

Other sounds may be produced if the heart is diseased or stressed. Rapid ventricular filling may cause a third heart sound early in diastole, a fourth sound may be heard when a forceful atrial contraction is required to fill a stiffened and diseased ventricle.

A triple rhythm may be produced due to extra sounds in diastole because of a stiff ventricular wall resisting filling. In fast heart rates this may be described as a *gallop* rhythm.

The opening of valves should not normally be audible, but the doctor may describe an opening snap heard as a rigid mitral valve opens. Ejection clicks may be heard as the pulmonary or aortic valves open if they are diseased.

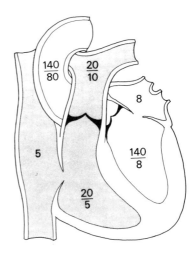

Fig. 2.7 Intracardiac pressures (in mmHg). Atrial pressures are the average mean pressures for the whole cardiac cycle.

MURMURS

Murmurs are heard due to the turbulent flow of blood through a narrow opening or due to an abnormally large flow of blood through an opening, be it a diseased valve or defective septum. These special sounds are best heard over particular parts of the heart or chest. The patient's cooperation will be needed to breathe quietly, to lean forward or to lie on their left side, and possibly to stop breathing for a few seconds while the doctor listens to the heart.

CARDIAC OUTPUT

The heart functions as a pump, giving an output of about five litres per minute in a resting adult. It contracts at a rate of about 70 beats per minute, ejecting a stroke volume of about 70 – 75 ml at each contraction.

Cardiac output (5 l) = rate (70/min) × stroke volume (72 ml)

During exercise or times of stress, the cardiac output can increase up to six times. This is achieved both by improving the contractile force of the ventricles to increase stroke volume and by raising the heart rate.

The tissues' demand for oxygenated blood is always changing so the cardiac output must vary accordingly. Many mechanisms affect cardiac output, and these will be discussed, but it must be remembered that at any one time several factors will be balancing each other to ensure that blood is delivered in the greatest quantity to those tissues that need it most, i.e. to the gut after a large meal or to the leg muscles while running, but always to the myocardium and brain.

CARDIAC INDEX

The larger the individual's body surface area (height × weight), the larger is the cardiac output needed to perfuse all the tissues. Therefore, to compare the cardiac output of different individuals, a cardiac index (litres/metre^2) or stroke index (ml/metre^2) is used when reporting on cardiological studies.

Regulation of cardiac output

Humoral and nervous information about the blood pressure, oxygenation, acidity, and temperature are relayed via receptors to the cardiac centre. The centre, which lies in the medulla oblongata, then regulates the heart rate and contractile force of the heart accordingly by balancing the autonomic nerves that supply the heart and blood vessels.

AUTONOMIC NERVOUS SYSTEM

The autonomic nervous system is made up of sympathetic and parasympathetic nerves. The vagus is the parasympathetic nerve that supplies the heart and it causes the sinus node to slow down during rest and sleep. The sympathetic system prepares the whole body for 'fight and flight'.

Sympathetic stimulation

Sympathetic stimulation has two main effects on the heart:
1 a *chronotropic* effect in that it speeds the sinus rate and atrio-ventricular conduction, and **2** an *inotropic* effect to increase muscle contractility. Both effects help to increase cardiac output in times of exercise or stress, but they also increase myocardial oxygen needs and irritability, which in the sick patient could cause angina and arrhythmias.

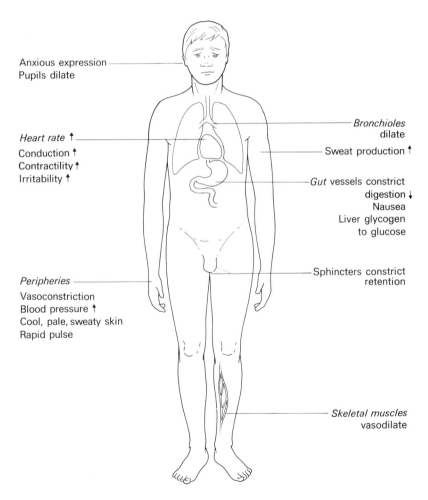

Anxious expression
Pupils dilate

Heart rate ↑
Conduction ↑
Contractility ↑
Irritability ↑

Bronchioles
dilate
Sweat production ↑

Gut vessels constrict
digestion ↓
Nausea
Liver glycogen
to glucose

Sphincters constrict
retention

Peripheries
Vasoconstriction
Blood pressure ↑
Cool, pale, sweaty skin
Rapid pulse

Skeletal muscles
vasodilate

Fig. 2.8 'Fight and flight' — effects of adrenaline and sympathetic stimulation.

Sympathetic stimulation is received by three types of receptors in the body: alpha, beta I and beta II. Alpha stimulation causes constriction of smooth muscle in all but heart or skeletal arterioles. Beta I stimulation causes chronotropic and inotropic cardiac effects. Beta II stimulation further prepares the body for 'fight and flight' by dilating bronchioles and skeletal muscle arterioles (Fig. 2.8).

The usual sympathetic postganglionic chemical transmitter is noradrenaline. The release of noradrenaline and adrenaline by the adrenal medulla further stimulates the heart to increase cardiac output and constrict arterioles to raise the blood pressure. The same occurs if intravenous adrenaline is given.

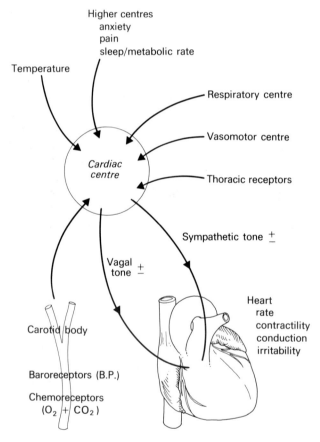

Fig. 2.9 The cardiac centre.

HIGHER CENTRES (Fig. 2.9)

The effect of the higher centres on the cardiac centre can be very marked; in anxious states the heart rate and force of contraction can double, e.g. before or during any stressful experience, including an examination in health, a race, pain, or any new procedure.

METABOLIC RATE

The raised metabolic rates found in thyrotoxicosis and fever increase cardiac output; deep sleep or hypothermia reduce heart rate and contractility. Temperature has an added direct effect on the sinus node and body temperature regulation involves the peripheral blood vessels. Heat is lost from the body when blood vessels near the skin are dilated; conversely in cold environments the body retains heat by the vasoconstriction of vessels in the skin and limb extremities.

BARORECEPTORS

Baroreceptors in the carotid arteries measure blood pressure. A rise in pressure would cause the vasomotor centre to increase vagal stimulation and reduce sympathetic tone so lowering heart rate, contractility and arteriolar constriction. Cardiac output and blood pressure would be reduced to normal levels. An increase in blood volume will, of course, increase venous return. A bigger venous return increases cardiac output, which in turn raises blood pressure, and this larger volume will stretch the aorta and carotid artery baroreceptors. Vasodilation (by a reduction in sympathetic tone) will accommodate the larger blood volume and return the blood pressure to normal.

CHEMORECEPTORS

Low oxygen and/or raised carbon dioxide (CO_2) levels will be measured by chemoreceptors in the aorta and carotid arteries. These then stimulate the respiratory centre, which in turn affects the cardiac centre to increase heart rate. This mechanism increases cardiac output to deliver more blood with fresh oxygen supplies to the tissues, and to increase CO_2 removal to the lungs which will also reduce pH. Notice that patients with respiratory distress have fast heart rates.

AUTOREGULATION

Working tissues will use oxygen and produce metabolites of carbon dioxide and lactic acid so that more blood will be needed in these areas than for resting tissues. In response to the CO_2 and metabolites, the autoregulatory system causes arterioles to working tissues to dilate, so providing more bloodflow to these areas.

In exercise and when there are other demands for greatly increased bloodflow, the resulting vasodilation from autoregulation will increase the rate at which blood flows from the arteries to the veins. Venous return to the heart will therefore be greatly increased.

VENOUS RETURN

Venous return is a most important factor in determining cardiac output. If the heart chambers are only filled with 50 ml, they can only eject a stroke volume of 50 ml. An increased venous return will stretch the atrium, this is relayed to the cardiac centre which will increase heart rate.

Contractility and Starling's law
The cardiac fibres can stretch to accommodate large volumes of blood. They have the unique property that the further they are stretched during diastole the more forcefully they will contract in systole, the heart can therefore eject into the arteries as much blood as returns via the veins, without 'damming back' blood and raising venous pressure. This increased contractility with a larger venous return is known as *Starling's law*. However, if the fibres become overstretched, only poor contraction occurs, the ventricles and veins become engorged with blood, cardiac output falls and exercise (with its resultant larger venous return) cannot be tolerated. Thus dyspnoea on exertion (due to raised pulmonary venous pressure) is common in those patients who have damaged heart muscle.

↑ concentration → ↓ 扩散 和 渗透

Diffusion and osmosis (Fig. 2.10)
The blood vessels, under the influence of sympathetic nerves, can vary in diameter to direct blood towards those tissues most in need. The semi-permeable membrane of the capillaries will then allow passage of nutrients to the tissues by diffusion and the return of wastes to the bloodstream by diffusion and osmosis. These methods rely on an intact capillary membrane, however the membrane can be damaged by toxins, extremes of temperature, or hypoxia.

Diffusion
Diffusion is the flow of fluid or gases from an area of high pressure to an area of low pressure. The blood pressure on the arterial side of a capillary is

higher than that within the interstitial space or on the venous side. The arterial pressure pushes the fluid with nutrients into the interstitial space that bathes the body cells. Oxygen also passes from the blood into areas of low oxygen concentration in the tissues; similarly carbon dioxide and other products of metabolism diffuse from the tissues into the lower CO_2 concentration of the blood to be taken to organs for detoxification and/or excretion.

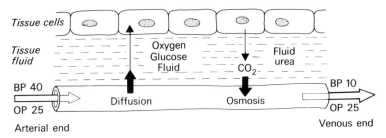

Fig. 2.10   Osmosis and diffusion between capillary blood and tissue cells. BP = blood pressure, OP = osmotic pressure — both in mmHg.

Osmosis

Osmosis is the flow of fluid through the semi-permeable membrane of the capillary wall, from an area of low concentration of particles in the interstitial fluid, to an area of high concentration of red cells and plasma proteins in the capillary. The large molecules of plasma proteins cannot leave the capillary and they exert an osmotic pressure. If these proteins are reduced, especially the albumen, the osmotic pressure will not be sufficient to draw all fluid back into the capillaries and interstitial oedema will result. Low albumen occurs with prolonged illness, malnutrition, and renal disease.

If the venous pressure is higher than the osmotic pressure, as can occur in venous obstruction or from the back pressure of heart failure, fluid will stay in the tissues in dependent parts of the body. Even healthy people who stand still for prolonged periods raise the pressure in the foot veins to as much as 13 kPa (90 mmHg). Aching, swollen legs may result, which recover on sitting or lying and resting the legs on a stool or bed.

Capillary shift mechanism and blood volume

An increased blood volume may be due to either an increased fluid intake or a reduced output. The increased volume of blood will stretch the capillaries, and more fluid will leave the circulation for the interstitial spaces by diffusion. A reduction in blood volume will have the opposite effect, causing increased re-absorption of fluid at the venous end of the capillary by osmosis. These mechanisms maintain a constant circulating blood volume and hence help to maintain cardiac output.

The muscle pump

To overcome the pull of gravity against the venous return the veins have one-way valves, which prevent blood flowing from the right heart back to the feet. Thus, on skeletal muscular contraction, the veins are squeezed and blood is pushed towards the heart. On exercise, the muscle pump action increases venous return which, as previously described, increases cardiac output (p. 34).

Raising the legs of a patient who is in shock and is hypovolaemic can greatly increase venous return and so improve cardiac output. To illustrate the importance of this, remember that even a healthy person may faint if they stand still for long periods, especially in a warm environment, because the leg veins will be engorged with blood and the lack of muscle action will reduce venous return to the extent that cardiac output will be inadequate to perfuse the brain. Repeated flexing of the leg muscles, even while standing still, will be enough to maintain venous return and prevent fainting. Leg exercises for the immobile patient are therefore of great importance to prevent stasis in the veins which may cause thrombosis to develop.

Intrathoracic pressure

Blood flows from an area of higher pressure in the arteries through the capillaries to the low pressure on the venous side. The pressure in the right atrium is equal to atmospheric pressure and is thus designated as 0 mm Hg.

The heart lies within the thoracic cage so that during inspiration when the thorax expands, a negative pressure of between -2 and -5 mmHg is created. The amount of blood flowing into the large thoracic veins and so to the heart will therefore increase. This negative phase is lost during positive pressure ventilation. Cardiac output may fall significantly when patients are ventilated.

Venous return from the head drains by gravity, the neck veins will be collapsed and not visible in health unless intrathoracic pressure is increased, as for example by straining at stool or by a singer sustaining a high note! Patients in longstanding cardiac failure often have a wasted appearance of their face and arms, with oedematous legs and abdomen but prominent neck veins.

The kidneys

The kidneys recognize and regulate changes in total circulating blood volume by increasing or reducing urine excretion. The kidneys also have a hormonal role, in that a low bloodflow or pressure to the kidneys causes renin to be secreted by the juxtaglomerular apparatus. This in turn activates circulating angiotensin to directly vasoconstrict the blood vessels in an effort to raise blood pressure to adequately perfuse the kidneys. A blood pressure of at least 11 – 13 kPa (80 – 90 mmHg) is necessary for filtration at Bowman's capsule (Fig. 2.11).

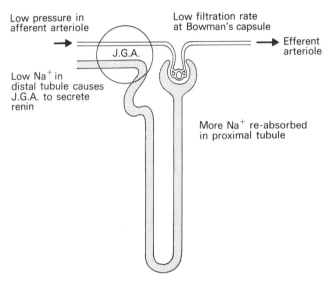

Fig. 2.11   Diagram to show the effects of reduced bloodflow in the kidneys (*see also* Table 2.1). JGA = Juxtaglomerular apparatus.

Aldosterone
This is another hormonal mechanism which raises circulating blood volume and hence blood pressure. Aldosterone is secreted by the adrenal cortex when the blood pressure falls, and is also triggered by the angiotensin mechanism. Aldosterone causes retention of salt by the kidney tubules and reduces the salt content of sweat, the higher sodium level in the blood raises blood osmolality so the pituitary gland excretes antidiuretic hormone to retain water in the distal renal tubules to dilute the salt with more body water. Blood volume is thereby increased.

BLOOD PRESSURE

The pressure of blood within the vessels depends on the diameter and length of the vessel, the elasticity of the arterial walls, the viscosity of the blood, the total blood volume, and the strength of myocardial contraction.

Blood pressure = total periphal resistance to flow × cardiac output

The systolic blood pressure indicates the maximum ejection pressure of the left ventricle at systole. The diastolic pressure will depend on the systolic pressure, the elasticity of the large arteries, peripheral resistance caused by arteriolar constriction, the viscosity of the blood, and the heart rate.

In the newborn, the artery walls are easily distended by a large volume of blood at only a low pressure. As age advances, the arteries become

Table 2.1   The effects of reduced bloodflow in the kidneys (*see also* Fig. 2.11).

Cause	Effect
Low BP in afferent arteriole	Low filtration rate at Bowman's capsule
Low filtration rate	More sodium re-absorbed in proximal tubule
Low sodium in distal tubule	JGA releases renin
Renin	Activates angiotensin
Angiotensin	BP increased by peripheral vasoconstriction to increase kidney bloodflow. Acts on adrenal glands to release aldosterone
Aldosterone	Acts on distal tubules to absorb more sodium. Salt content of sweat increased
Increased blood sodium	Raises blood osmolality which stimulates the pituitary
Pituitary	Releases antidiuretic hormone
ADH	Acts on kidneys to re-absorb more water to maintain normal osmolality
Increased water	Increases blood volume and preload. Ventricles are stretched thus increasing cardiac output (Starling's law)
Increased blood volume	Increased venous pressure leading to peripheral oedema and liver congestion

harder to the extreme that those with arteriosclerosis have inelastic calcified arteries that cannot distend at systole, or recoil during diastole.

Regulation of blood pressure is by varying the peripheral resistance (Fig. 2.12), brought about by the vasomotor centre controlling blood vessel size, and by other factors that affect cardiac output (Fig. 2.9).

The medulla oblongata helps to control these variables by balancing autonomic nerve impulse to the heart and blood vessels in conjunction with the neighbouring cardiac centre. As seen on page 32, sympathetic beta I activity has a chronotropic and inotropic effect to increase cardiac output, and alpha stimulation causes arteriolar vasoconstriction. The vasomotor centre receives information from the baroreceptors in the aorta and carotid arteries which relay the degree of stretch caused by ventricular systole. The centre will then increase or decrease alpha stimulation accordingly.

chronotropic drug $+$ ↑ HR
$-$ ↓ HR

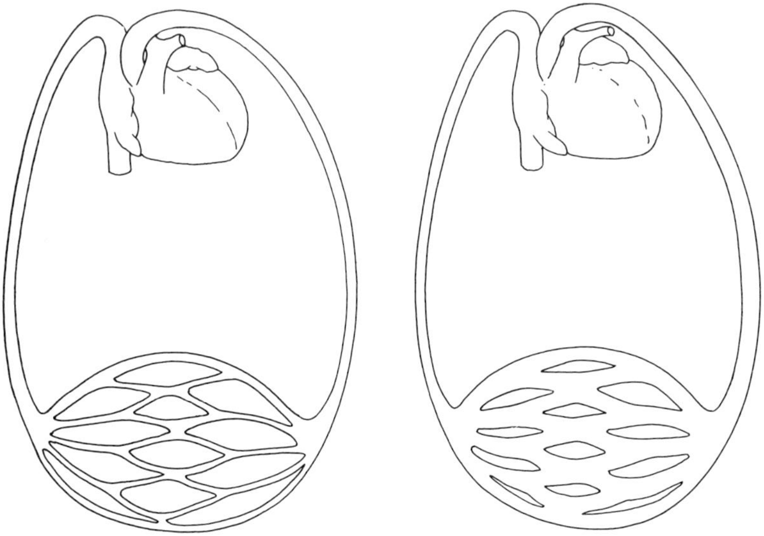

High peripheral resistance   Low peripheral resistance

Fig. 2.12 The mechanism of peripheral vascular resistance. With high peripheral resistance, flow drops, ejection becomes more difficult, pressure rises and there is an increased afterload; with low peripheral resistance, flow rises, ejection is easier, pressure drops and afterload is reduced.

Peripheral resistance (see Fig. 2.12)
The relaxation or constriction of blood vessels will re-distribute the flow of blood to tissues most in need. It does this either by autoregulation or as a result of the vasomotor centre altering sympathetic tone in response to various body receptors (p. 32).

The body is normally maintained in slight sympathetic tone, but should strong alpha stimulation occur, vasoconstriction of all but heart and skeletal muscle arterioles results. This vasoconstriction increases blood pressure and the resistance against which the heart must pump. This resistance to cardiac ejection is called afterload. An increase in peripheral vascular resistance increases afterload and requires the left heart to work harder. An increase in pulmonary vascular resistance, i.e. afterload of the right heart, requires the right heart to work harder.

To maintain the cardiac output in the presence of a greater afterload, the heart must work harder by improving myocardial contractility. The blood pressure will rise, but tissue perfusion and cardiac output will not necessarily change.

In the presence of a reduced cardiac output, sympathetic stimulation produces vasoconstriction to maintain blood pressure. The patient in impending shock will initially maintain his blood pressure, even though he is pale, anxious, and tachycardic with a reduced urine output and cool, sweaty peripheries. Should the blood pressure then begin to fall, this is a late and serious sign.

When sudden peripheral vasoconstriction occurs, e.g. to prevent loss of body heat on leaving a warm house on a cold day, or on taking a cold shower after exercise, the tremendous increase in afterload will demand the heart to work harder. This increase in afterload could prove too much heart work for a patient with a diseased or ischaemic heart. Angina or acute left ventricular failure could occur.

Cardiac output × peripheral resistance = blood pressure.

On the other hand, vasodilation reduces peripheral resistance and consequently makes it easier for the left ventricle to eject blood into the aorta. Glyceryl trinitrate causes widespread vasodilation and hence reduces afterload, heart work, and oxygen consumption — thus relieving angina.

If vasodilation is excessive, as occurs in anaphylactic or septicaemic shock, the blood pressure will fall to dangerous levels in spite of an increase in cardiac output. Venous return will fall (as ascertained by a low CVP) and, unless the patient is rapidly transfused with blood or plasma, the cardiac output will fall, so that blood pressure to even vital centres will be inadequate to sustain life.

It can be seen that cardiac output, peripheral resistance, blood pressure and venous return are linked and dependent on one another. Should one factor be impaired or inappropriate, the others will try to compensate to maintain perfusion of at least the essential organs.

Chapter 3
Electrocardiography and arrhythmias

THE ELECTROCARDIOGRAM (ECG) RECORDING

The ECG is a recording of the changing voltages between cardiac muscle. The body is an excellent conductor of these changing potentials because it is largely composed of fluid and electrolytes. In addition, if the skin is clean there is little resistance to the current flow through electrodes placed on the skin surface.

The electrical waveforms produced by the changing voltages are burnt with a hot stylus or drawn with ink onto graph paper, and can be displayed on a screen. The characteristic wave forms of PQRST represent the varying electrical activity of impulses passing through the atria, conducting system, and ventricles (Fig. 3.1). A flat line, the isoelectric line, indicates that no changes in voltage are taking place.

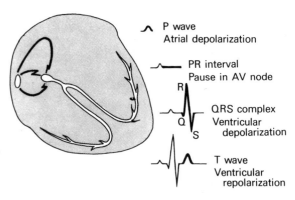

Fig. 3.1 The conducting system and how the PQRST complex is associated with it.

The best method to learn the normal duration of each wave and segment is to relate the wave produced on the ECG to the physiological happenings within the heart. A good knowledge of the normal durations is essential for anyone wishing to interpret ECG tracings (Fig. 3.2).

42

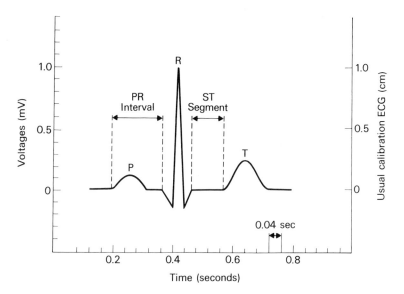

Fig. 3.2   The nomenclature and measurement of normal ECG deflections on the graph paper.

P. WAVE

The relationship between the P waves, if any, and the QRS complexes is the key to arrhythmia interpretation. P waves should be present, of the same shape as each other, and precede each QRS complex in a regular fashion. The height of the P wave should be no more than 3 mm in bipolar leads or 2 – 5 mm in unipolar leads and no wider than 0.1 seconds.

P waves may vary in the following fashion: **1**   A tall P wave is called *P pulmonale*, and indicates right atrial enlargement and strain due to a high pulmonary vascular resistance. This can be caused by pulmonary disease, pulmonary valve stenosis, or left heart disease. **2**   A wide P wave indicates left atrial strain, usually due to mitral valve disease, so-called *P mitrale*, it is often notched. **3**   P waves prior to premature QRS complexes or tachycardias may be inverted or otherwise different from the underlying rhythm and give the clue to the origin of the abnormal rhythm. **4**   P waves of premature or blocked beats may be hidden in the QRS complex or T wave of preceding complexes, the T wave and ST segments should be closely examined and compared. **5**   P waves may be absent in junctional rhythm or sinoatrial block, or may be replaced by fibrillation or flutter waves.

PR INTERVAL

The PR interval is normally 0.1 – 0.2 seconds in duration. It should be a constant measurement in the individual patient, at a given heart rate: the faster the heart rate, the shorter the PR interval. Any change in PR interval indicates a change in conduction between the atria and bundle branches.

QRS DURATION

If the distance between the first and last deflection of the QRS complex is longer than 0.1 seconds, then a defect or block to conduction exists in the bundle branches.

ST SEGMENT

The ST segment is usually 0.14 – 0.16 seconds in duration. This will follow the QRS complex and, in health, is isoelectric. If depressed or elevated it is an indication of ischaemia or injury due, for example, to coronary artery disease.

QT INTERVAL

The QT interval is usually 0.33 – 0.43 seconds in duration. This measurement is important because a prolonged QT interval increases the vulnerable period and the likelihood of ectopics causing ventricular fibrillation, particularly post-infarction or with quinidine-type drugs, e.g. disopyramide (*see* p. 28).

T WAVE

A T wave will always follow a QRS complex. Innumerable variables will alter its shape. These include ischaemia, drugs (notably digoxin and quinidine-type drugs), hypothermia, hyperkalaemia, change in heart rates and hypertension. The T wave may be upright, peaked, inverted or flattened, symmetrical or asymmetrical. Changes due to potassium or ischaemia are the most important for the nurse to consider. The T wave is usually not taller than 5 mm in standard leads, or 10 mm in precordial leads.

U WAVE

This wave may be seen following the T wave in bradycardia, in patients on digoxin therapy or those with hypokalaemia. Its significance is not known.

P wave   No higher than 2.5 mm or wider than 0.1 seconds
PR interval   0.1 – 0.2 seconds
QRS duration   0.07 – 0.1 seconds

If these normal values in conduction time of the impulse are exceeded, there is some block or partial block in the special conducting fibres, e.g. if the PR interval is prolonged over 0.22 seconds, the AV node is conducting the impulse slowly from the atria to the bundle branches. This is called 1st degree block (Fig. 3.3) and may be due to ischaemia, drugs, injury, or fibrosis. Likewise if the QRS duration is prolonged, one of the bundle branches is not functioning. This is called bundle branch block (Fig. 3.4). Note the QRS is wide over 0.12 seconds. The 12 lead ECG must be examined to diagnose which of the bundles is blocked.

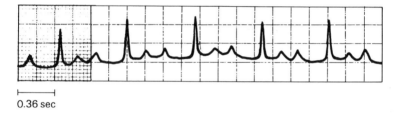

0.36 sec

Fig. 3.3   First degree AV block. The PR interval is 0.36 seconds.

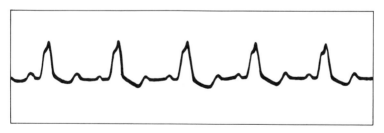

Fig. 3.4   Bundle branch block. The QRS interval is more than 0.12 seconds.

Should the sinus node fail, or its impulse be blocked, other areas of the heart can take over as pacemaker, but they will initiate the impulses more slowly, and less reliably than the sinus node (Fig. 3.5) (*see also* action potential, p. 26). That is, if the sinus node fails to initiate an impulse, the atrioventricular node may do so, sending impulses down the bundles and Purkinje fibres equally to both ventricles. In this case, the ECG will show normal QRS complexes but no P waves (Fig. 3.6) — a junctional rhythm. If both sinus and AV node fail to send impulses to the ventricles, some ventricular cells may initiate the impulse, producing a slower rate — a ventricular escape rhythm.

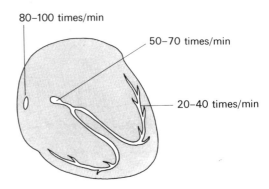

Fig. 3.5 Intrinsic depolarization times of the sinus node, AV node, and ventricles.

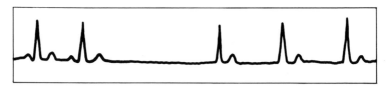

Fig. 3.6 ECG of (*left*) sinus rhythm,(*centre*) sinus arrest, and (*right*) junctional escape rhythm.

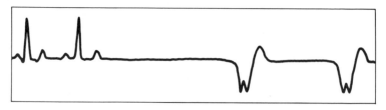

Fig. 3.7 ECG as above, but with ventricular escape beats.

In Figure 3.7, notice how wide and bizarre the ventricular escape QRS is. This is because impulses have come from a site (focus) within the ventricles and spread slowly to other muscle cells — not using the specialized conducting pathways.

The 12 lead ECG

The duration of each wave and segment, discussed above, can be measured from any set of electrodes placed over the heart and will indicate how well the main conducting pathways are working, i.e. the cardiac rhythm.

The 12 lead ECG uses 12 sets of electrodes to assess how 12 different areas of cardiac muscle are conducting impulses. The strength and direction of impulses gives shape and size to the Q, R and S waves recorded in these areas, which can be compared to known normals to build a picture of health or disease, e.g. the death or hypertrophy of a particular portion of cardiac muscle.

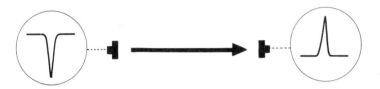

Fig. 3.8 Relationship of impulse direction to ECG deflection.

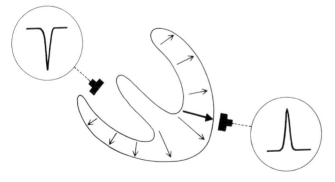

Fig. 3.9 Movement of impulses from the endocardium to the epicardium.

READING THE 12 LEAD ECG

The changing potentials within the heart that create the electrical impulses will sometimes be travelling towards where the electrodes have been placed, and sometimes away, depending on the timing of the cardiac cycle and the thickness of the heart muscle under the electrode. Any impulse travelling towards an electrode will give an upright *positive* deflection (Fig. 3.8). Any impulse travelling away from an electrode will give a downward or *negative* deflection.

The impulses activate the endocardium from the Purkinje fibres. The impulses then spread towards the epicardium, i.e. from inside out (Fig. 3.9). The ECG picks out the main vector (Fig. 3.10), which is a sum of all impulses occurring at that time. A vector shows with an arrow the main direction of the depolarization impulse. The size of the arrows show how forceful the depolarization wave is. A large depolarization wave could be due to either a thickened myocardium or a delay in depolarization time, e.g. due to conduction problems, such as bundle branch block.

Fig. 3.10 A vector derived from two impulses of different duration and strength.

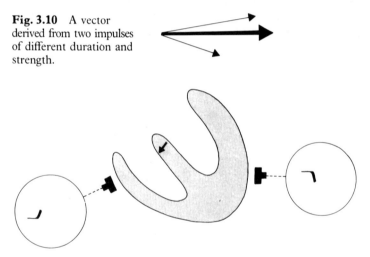

Fig. 3.11 The septal vector in a normal heart.

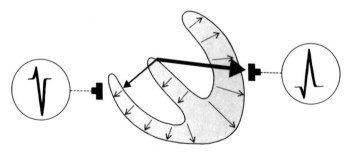

Fig. 3.12 The main ventricular depolarization vector in a normal heart.

In a healthy adult the left ventricle is many times thicker than the right ventricle. The septum likewise is mostly left ventricular muscle, so the septal depolarization wave occurs from inside the left ventricle, i.e. from left to right, and the main ventricular vector points towards the thicker left ventricle (Figs. 3.11 & 3.12).

AXIS

Knowledge of the direction of the main vector gives information concerning the thickness of the ventricular walls, which might change with hypertrophy or death of myocardium (Figs. 3.13 & 3.14) (myocardial infarction). This dead muscle is electrically silent so does not contribute to the vector force or direction. In this case the electrical axis of the heart will be said to shift. The axis also appears abnormal if the heart is lying on its side (as in short fat people) or lying more vertical than usual (as in tall thin people), even though the main vector will in fact be pointing normally

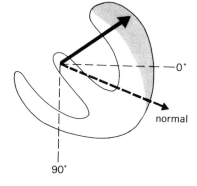

Fig. 3.13 The main ventricular vector in left ventricular hypertrophy showing left axis deviation.

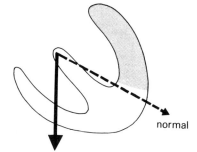

Fig. 14 The shift in the ventricular vector axis away from infarcted myocardium.

towards their thicker left ventricle. The axis of the main vector can be plotted as described on p. 54.

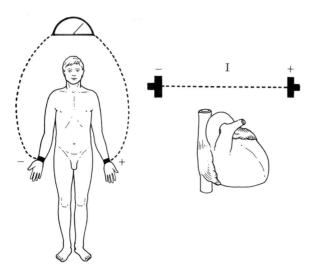

Fig. 3.15   Placement of lead I — positive pole to left arm.

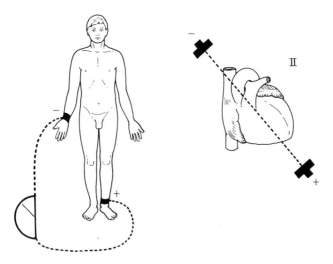

Fig. 3.16   Placement of lead II — positive pole to left leg.

THE 12 LEADS

To determine the direction of these main vectors, the impulses are recorded on a 12 lead ECG. In 1901, Einthoven first recorded three leads on a string galvanometer. These three leads were bipolar having a negative and a positive pole (Figs. 3.15 – 3.17). As described above, any impulse going towards the positive pole would give a positive or upright deflection.

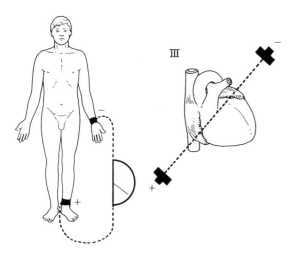

Fig. 3.17 Placement of lead III — positive pole to left leg.

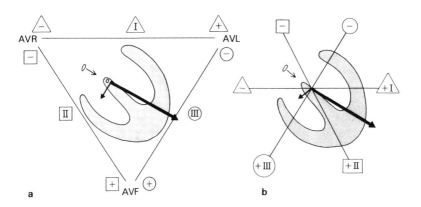

Fig. 3.18 The heart and main vectors within Einthoven's triangle (*left*) and within the triaxial reference system derived from this (*right*).

In Einthoven's triangle the heart is electrically central (Fig. 3.18). The ECG machine is wired for the three standard limb leads as shown in Fig. 3.18 where three main points are apparent:

1 The P wave vector is parallel in lead II and travelling towards its

positive pole so that the P wave is usually more clearly seen in lead II.
2 The septal vector will be negative in lead I, not seen in lead II (as it is
vertical to it), and positive in lead III.
3 The main QRS vector will usually be positive in three standard limb
leads, but may be small in lead III as it is almost vertical to it (i.e. travelling
neither towards nor away from the pole).

Wilson (1933) added three unipolar leads: right arm, left arm and left
leg. Any impulse travelling towards these electrodes will be positive and
any impulse travelling away will be negative. The size of these leads is
augmented on all ECG machines to make voltages of comparable size to
the limb leads and so aid interpretation.

The leads are called augmented vector, right, left, or foot (AVR, AVL,
AVF). You should note also that AVR is called a cavity lead, because it
looks into the heart and so only sees impulses travelling outwards towards
the epicardium. For this reason it is usually negative. AVL is similar to
lead I and usually positive. AVF is similar to leads II and III and is also
usually positive.

Fig. 3.19 shows the triaxial reference system and Fig. 3.20 shows the
hexaxial reference systems. These reference systems are used to plot the
axis of the main ventricular vector. In the normal ECG with the heart
lying normally in the thorax, the main vector will be between 0° and + 90°
(Figs. 3.13 & 3.20b). If the vector lies between –30° and –120° left axis
deviation exists, if the vector lies between +90°and 180°, right axis
deviation is present.

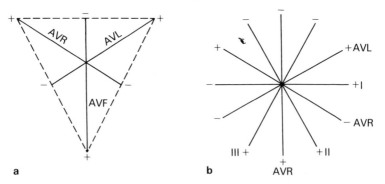

a

b   AVR

Fig. 3.19   (*Left*) The triaxial reference system formed by the unipolar extremity
leads. (*Right*) The combination of the triaxial reference system of the standard and
unipolar leads to form a hexaxial reference system.

Perhaps the easiest leads of the 12-lead ECG for the nurse to remember
are the chest leads. The positions of leads V1 – V6 can be seen to reflect

changes in the septal, anterior, and lateral aspect of the heart (Fig. 3.21).

Lead V1 is placed over the 4th intercostal space, one inch (2.5 cm) to the right of the sternum.

Lead V2 is also placed over the 4th intercostal space, but one inch (2.5 cm) to the left of the sternum.

Lead V3 is placed between lead V2 and lead V4.

Lead V4 is placed in the mid-clavicular line of the 5th intercostal space.

Lead V5 is placed in the anterior axillary line at the same level as lead V4.

Lead V6 is placed in the mid-axillary line, again at the same level as lead V4.

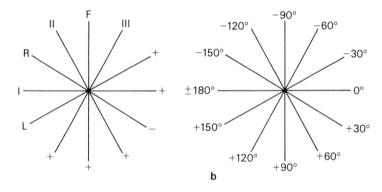

Fig. 3.20 The hexaxial reference system.

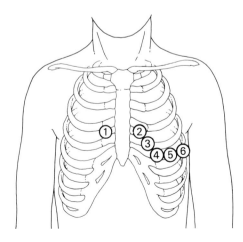

Fig. 3.21 Position of chest leads for ECG recording.

Progression of the R wave through the V leads

The R wave increases in height from being very small in V1 to being very tall in V6. Similarly the S wave is very deep in V1 and it gradually becomes smaller throughout the V leads, until it is almost invisable in lead V6 (Fig. 3.22).

The small R wave in V1 is very important because it represents the septal vector (*see* Fig. 3.11), the deep S wave is the negative deflection caused by the large left ventricular vector going away from the V1 electrode. Likewise there is a small Q wave at the beginning of V6 representing the septal depolarization; the tall R wave of V6 and the other left ventricular leads is due to the main QRS vector travelling towards them.

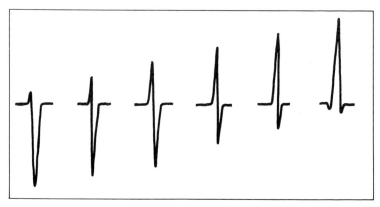

Fig. 3.22   Progression of the R wave through chest leads.

MEASURING THE QRS AXIS

There are two methods to approximately determine the mean QRS axis.

Method 1

Look at the 12 lead ECG (Fig. 3.23), find a lead with a biphasic QRS or the lead with the smallest complex. In this example use AVL, which is biphasic, and study its axis on the reference system. The mean QRS axis is neither going towards nor away from the positive pole of AVL. It is at right angles to it.

The lead with its axis at right angles to AVL is lead II and, in Fig. 3.23, lead II has a large positive deflection. The main QRS vector is therefore going towards the positive pole of lead II. This will give a normal axis of 60° (Fig. 3.24).

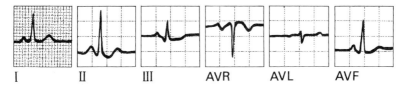

Fig. 3.23   Normal 12 lead ECG.

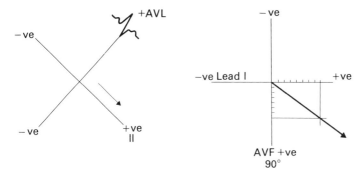

Fig. 3.24   (*Left*) One way of measuring the QRS axis. (*Right*) An alternative way of measuring the direction of the main QRS vector.

Method 2

The axes of lead I and lead AVF cross each other at right angles on the hexaxial reference system (Fig. 3.20). Draw these two leads and mark in their positive and negative poles. Lead I (in Fig. 3.23) is eight small squares tall on the ECG paper, so mark the axis 8 mm towards the positive pole on lead I. The R wave in lead AVF is also eight squares tall in this example but AVL has a one square negative Q wave as well; so mark 7 mm towards the positive pole of lead AVF. Now bisect the angle to find the direction of the mean QRS vector (Fig. 3.20).

Bundle branch block

The bundle of His divides into *three* distinct fascicles, the right bundle, the left anterior bundle, and the left posterior bundle branch. The left posterior fascicle divides proximally from the bundle of His and activates the posterior and inferior parts of the left ventricle. The left anterior fascicle activates anterior and lateral parts of the left ventricle.

Should one of two fascicles block, the patient will be unaware, and his monitor will continue to show sinus rhythm, but with a widened QRS complex. Many fully fit people are found to have bundle branch block (BBB) on routine ECG examination. In this case, heart sounds will be affected and ECG diagnosis of myocardial infarction or disease will be more complex. If a 12 lead ECG is examined it shows, most clearly in the V leads, that the part of the heart muscle usually activated by the blocked bundle will have delayed depolarization (Fig. 3.25). This will result in the mean QRS vector shifting to that side: left bundle branch block results in left axis deviation and right bundle branch block results in right axis deviation (Figs. 3.26 & 3.27). The causes are the same as for AV block (p. 75).

A common finding in elderly people, right BBB can be congenital, but left BBB is a more serious finding as it may indicate ischaemic heart disease.

BIFASCICULAR BLOCK

The significance of BBB to the patient and to the nurse is that all three fascicles could block to cause ventricular standstill (cardiac arrest). Like atrioventricular block, bundle branch block may gradually progress from the patient being asymptomatic and in no danger to being in asystole. The bifascicular block can be recognized by a change in the QRS axis due to delayed activation of another distinct portion of the myocardium. The QRS pattern on the monitor will change and this should alert the nurse to record a 12 lead ECG, which should be compared to previous 12 lead ECGs. The following features may be apparent.

Right bundle branch block with left posterior hemiblock
   = RBBB pattern but increased left axis deviation
      lead AVL shows:
         small Q wave
         tall R wave
         delayed intrinsicoid deflection
         notched R wave
         secondary T wave changes
Right bundle branch block with left posterior hemiblock
   = RBBB with right axis deviation
      S wave in lead I and tall R wave in leads II, III and AVF
      lead II shows:
         small Q wave
         tall R wave
         delayed intrinsicoid deflection
         notched R wave
         secondary T wave changes.

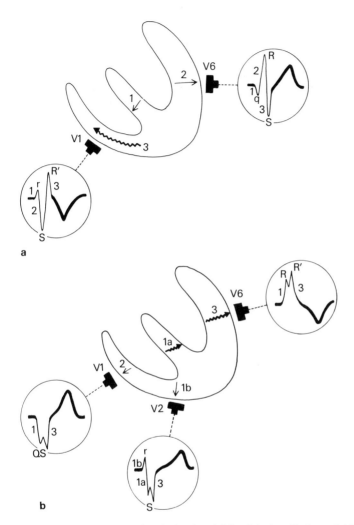

Fig. 3.25 Ventricular depolarization (**a**) in right bundle branch block and its effect on V1 and V6, (**b**) in left bundle branch block and its effect on V1, V2, and V6.

NURSING INTERVENTION FOR BBB

The nursing intervention will depend on the patient's present illness and recent history. A history of *Stokes – Adams attacks* indicates that all three fascicles occasionally block to cause periods of ventricular standstill. The patient should be nursed within view and monitored if possible. A 12 lead

ECG should be taken and carefully examined, and the doctor notified immediately the patient arrives on the ward. An intravenous line may be established and temporary transvenous pacemaker insertion arranged as soon as possible to prevent a fatal Stokes-Adams attack occurring.

Following recent *myocardial infarction* the development of BBB may indicate infarction extension. The patient should be asked if he is experiencing pain, and his general condition should be assessed. A 12 lead ECG should be taken, examined and the doctor notified. If the ECG reveals that two of the three fascicles of the bundle branch system are blocked, the patient should be closely observed in case the final bundle blocks causing complete block and ventricular standstill. Temporary transvenous pacing will be considered.

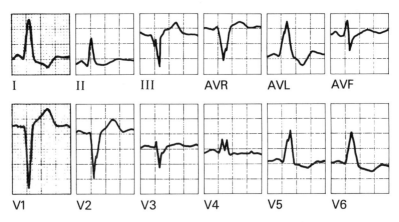

Fig. 3.26   ECG showing left bundle branch block. Note (a) the M-shaped QRS complex in left ventricular leads — well seen in lead V4 but barely discernible in leads V5 and V6; and (b) the broad QS complex in the right ventricular leads — leads V1 and V2. The QRS duration is 0.12 seconds (three small squares).

ARRHYTHMIAS

The term arrhythmia literally means 'no rhythm' but is used to describe any abnormal rhythm. Another term commonly used is dysrrhythmia.

We have already discussed how the heart beat is normally initiated by an impulse from the sinus node, which is then conducted through the atrioventricular node to both ventricles and results in sinus rhythm, with a regular apex and pulse rate. We have also briefly mentioned (p. 46) that when the sinus node fails or the AV node blocks its impulses, then other cardiac tissue will take over as the pacemaker at a slower rate. All cardiac tissue has the capacity for automatic depolarization, but this capacity is best developed in the sinus node. If other areas of the heart depolarize automatically ahead of the sinus node, this results in tachycardias or extra premature beats, called ectopics. The site of this early depolarizing heart tissue is called an ectopic focus. It may be in the atria, AV node, or ventricles; the shape of the ectopic QRS on the ECG and its relationship to any P waves will indicate the site of its origin.

IRRITABILITY

Following myocardial infarction or cardiac surgery not only do cells that were predominantly contractile become pacemaker cells, but the threshold for automatic depolarization is lowered, encouraging ectopic foci to develop and depolarize ahead of the sinus node. The heart then is said to be more irritable. Other factors that increase this irritability are hypoxia, acidosis, raised carbon dioxide, low serum potassium, diminished coronary bloodflow, circulating catecholamines, and most inotropic drugs. A bradycardia may encourage an ectopic escape rhythm, which could be undesirable in an irritable heart.

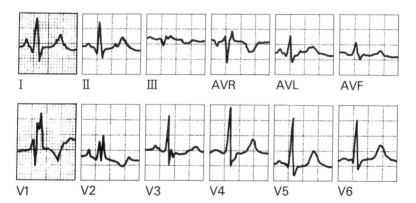

Fig. 3.27   ECG showing right bundle branch block. Note (a) the M-shaped QRS complex in the right ventricular leads — V1 and V2; and (b) the delayed and slurred S wave in the left ventricular leads — V4 to V6.

THE VULNERABLE PERIOD OR R ON T PHENOMENON

If an electrical stimuli were applied to the heart during the QRS complex, there would be no response as the heart would be completely refractory. At other times in the cardiac cycle, where the heart is completely repolarized, a stimulus would cause a single ectopic beat.

The T wave on the ECG represents the repolarization process. During this time the heart is partly refractory and partly repolarized. This period is called the vulnerable period, because any impulse landing on the top of the T wave could cause repetitive ectopic formation to give ventricular tachycardia or fatal ventricular fibrillation.

Following myocardial infarction, and probably following cardiac surgery, the QT interval is lengthened and the vulnerable period is extended to the full width of the T wave. This increases the risk of ventricular fibrillation from any ectopic beat that falls soon after the preceding QRS. For this reason cardioversion for atrial arrhythmias is synchronized to the patient's cardiac cycle, so that the impulse falls within the QRS complex, when the ventricles are totally refractory.

PROGNOSTIC IMPLICATIONS

Most arrhythmias will not disturb the patient at all and may be of no consequence, therefore they require no treatment. Other rhythm changes may herald more serious or life-threatening arrhythmias, for example, R on T phenomenon, and some rhythms may cause or precipitate heart failure, for example, atrial fibrillation. A knowledge of the different arrhythmias, and how to recognize them is therefore useful. Recognition of the compensatory mechanisms and haemodynamic effects the rhythm is having on the individual patient will also indicate when treatment is required.

HAEMODYNAMIC EFFECTS

If the heart rate is too fast or too slow, cardiac output will be impaired. Patients with severe cardiac disease or post-infarction or cardiac surgery may develop sudden and severe symptoms of shock with vasoconstriction, hypotension, dizziness, blurring of vision, or loss of consciousness. For patients with less severe heart disease, the inappropriate rate will produce ventricular strain and heart failure over a period of days or weeks.

The completely irregular rhythm of atrial fibrillation may cause a 30% drop in cardiac output, due to loss of effective atrial contraction plus the irregular and inconsistent filling of the ventricles prior to their erratically timed contraction. In junctional rhythms, or ventricular paced rhythms, the rhythm will be regular so that, although atrial contraction is lost, cardiac output will probably be well maintained. Treatment will therefore depend on the patient's symptoms as well as the ECG rhythm.

Calculating the rhythm rate (see Fig. 3.2)
If the rhythm is regular, i.e. the RR and PP intervals are constant, the ventricular and atrial rates can be calculated accurately by counting the number of squares between the RR or PP interval. Divide the number of small squares into 1500, or the larger squares into 300, to establish the heart rate. A less accurate method is to count the number of R waves on a 150 cm (6 inch) strip and multiply by 10 to establish the rate per minute.

Sinus bradycardia   — *Arpine*

Rhythm	regular
Rate	less than 60 per minute
P waves	one present before each QRS complex
PR interval	normal
QRS duration	normal

It is evident that this rhythm originates in a slowly firing sinus node (Fig. 3.28). Normal conduction occurs through the AV node (normal PR interval) and within the bundle branches and ventricles (normal QRS duration).

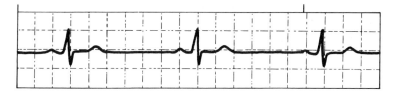

Fig. 3.28   Sinus bradycardia.

CAUSES

Drugs such as beta blocking agents or digoxin may be involved (although other arrhythmias or symptoms are usually evident). There may be increased vagal tone from severe pain, neurogenic shock and inferior myocardial ischaemia or infarction. Sinus node disease may cause alternating bradycardias and tachycardias. Athletic persons' hearts are capable of large stroke volumes; therefore, at rest, the rate is slow.

Non-cardiac causes include hypothermia, myxoedema, and raised intracranial pressure.

NURSING INTERVENTION

This will depend on the patient's general condition and the symptoms.

Usually the patient will be asymptomatic unless he has a reduced cardiac reserve. If he is hypotensive or dizzy, lay him down and elevate the legs to increase venous return. This will raise the stroke volume and cardiac output. If the patient is dyspnoeic, position him head and feet up by jack-knifing the bed or using pillows. Stay with the patient until symptoms pass.

To identify and document the rhythm, record an ECG tracing; the apex, not the pulse, should be recorded. A slow pulse rate could be due to heart block, ectopic beats, or sinus arrest which are more sinister than sinus bradycardia. Notify the medical staff immediately if the patient experiences any symptoms or escape rhythms.

TREATMENT

Atropine 0.6 – 1.2 mg i.v. increases the sinus node rate by blocking the vagus nerve. Isoprenaline or adrenaline may be given by infusion if the bradycardia persists or is extreme. Pacing, either temporary or permanent, may be indicated. Drugs that induce bradycardias should be reduced or stopped and serum digoxin levels should be estimated if toxicity is suspected. If severe pain is the cause, diamorpine 2 – 5 mg i.v. should be given along with atropine.

Sinus arrhythmia

Rhythm   irregular, speeds and slows in a regular fashion
Rate   between 60 and 100 per minute
P waves   present and identical before each QRS complex
PR interval   constant
QRS duration   narrow

Rhythm originates in the sinus node and is normally conducted via the AV node and the bundle branches, but the sinus node is firing in an irregular pattern.

Notice also the patient's respiratory pattern since the rate usually speeds with inspiration and slows with expiration due to stretch receptors in the lungs stimulating the vagus nerve. Sinus arrhythmia is common in children and the elderly, and patients are usually asymptomatic.

NURSING INTERVENTION

No nursing action is necessary, except to clearly identify that the cause of the irregular pulse in a sick patient is due to sinus arrhythmia, not atrial fibrillation or ectopic beats. To do this, record an ECG tracing.

TREATMENT

None necessary, except during the slower phases if there are escape ventricular ectopics in the post-infarction or cardiac surgery patient. Atropine 0.6 – 1.2 mg should speed the sinus rate and abolish ectopics.

Sinus tachycardia

The PQRST sequence in sinus tachycardia is similar to sinus rhythm, but the rate is faster.

CAUSES

These include sympathetic stimulation, fear, pain, anxiety, exercise (though the rate should slow with rest), fever, heart failure, thyrotoxicosis, hypovolaemia, tamponade, and drugs, e.g. adrenaline, isoprenaline, atropine, aminophylline.

NURSING INTERVENTION

Assess the patient's general condition, identify any of the above causes, and treat as appropriate.

Supraventricular tachycardias (SVT)

This condition covers any tachycardia that is not ventricular in origin, including atrial tachycardia, junctional tachycardia, and fast atrial fibrillation or flutter.

The QRS complexes are so close together when the heart is beating very fast (160–210 beats per minute) that it is almost impossible to identify these tachycardias apart. The regularity and the relationship of the P wave to the QRS complex gives the clue to the rhythm, but this may be hidden in the QRS complex or T wave of the preceding or following beat.

The patient's symptoms and management are similar, but attempts should be made to identify the origin of the rhythm to aid specific treatment. The beginning or the end of a run of SVT can give the clue. Sometimes the rhythm will come and go in short bursts, or may last for hours.

NURSING INTERVENTION FOR VERY FAST HEART RATES

Put the patient comfortably to bed. Assess the general condition while observing the heart rate and rhythm. Notice if there are other signs or symptoms of pain, breathlessness or dizziness which either precipitated or follow the attack. Stay with the patient and notify the medical staff. Record a monitor rhythm tracing or a 12 lead ECG if possible.

TREATMENT

An increase in vagal tone may slow the rhythm or convert it to sinus rhythm. Tone may be increased by eyeball pressure, carotid sinus massage, or the Valsalva manoeuvre (*see* p. 104). Occasionally asystole will occur with an increase in vagal tone.

Drugs
Slow intravenous administration of the following drugs may revert or slow the rhythm practolol 5 – 10 mg, disopyramide 50 – 100 mg, verapamil 5 – 10 mg, digoxin 0 – 5 mg. The latter three may then be given orally.

Cardioversion (see p. 143)
A direct current electrical shock, synchronized to the patient's ECG and applied across the heart, may be used immediately if the patient is severely haemodynamically embarrassed by the tachycardia. Cardioversion may be used for tachycardias that are resistant to drugs, but should not be used on patients receiving digoxin.

Overpacing
For patients who experience recurrent tachycardia, a pacemaker may be inserted so that, when a tachycardia does occur, a few impulses are delivered at the rate of 200 – 400/minute to capture and depolarize the atria. (This can also be used to treat ventricular tachycardia.) Since the sinus node is normally the fastest tissue to repolarize, sinus rhythm can be re-established in much the same way as cardioversion, but without the necessity of frequent and unpleasant shocks.

Atrial tachycardia (Fig. 3.29)

Rhythm	P waves regular
	RR intervals equal except for one on Fig. 3.29
P waves	numerous ectopic atrial P waves
PR intervals	variable
QRS	of normal duration

This rhythm is due to excitable atria; a varying AV block is present but, if a 1:1 conduction was present, the ventricular rate would be over 200 and cause severe symptoms.

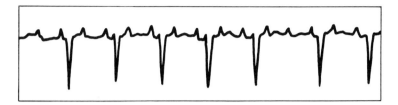

Fig. 3.29   Atrial tachycardia.

CAUSES

This may occur post-infarction or cardiac surgery, but also in healthy individuals who will experience episodes of palpitations, breathlessness and dizziness — paroxysmal atrial tachycardia.

Atrial fibrillation (Fig. 3.30)

Rhythm	irregularly irregular
P waves	none clearly distinguishable, but many small irregular waves visible on the base line
Rate	the atria bombard the AV node with up to 600 impulses per minute, the number that are conducted to the ventricles will determine the ventricular rate. This may vary from very slow to very fast.
QRS duration	normal
Pulse	due to the irregular time for the heart to fill and contract, QRS complexes that occur closely behind another beat will not give a large enough stroke volume to cause a pulse. The apex will be faster than the pulse rate

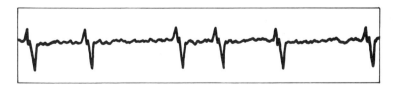

Fig. 3.30   Atrial fibrillation.

CAUSES

These include ischaemic heart disease, heart failure, rheumatic valve disease, thyrotoxic heart disease, or can be idiopathic. Digoxin toxicity can also cause rapid atrial fibrillation.

NURSING INTERVENTION

Assess the effect of the rate and irregularity on the particular patient. If he is asymptomatic, document and mention this rhythm change to medical staff. If he has symptoms such as palpitations, chest pain, breathlessness or dizziness, notify the medical staff and rest the patient.

This rhythm often reverts to sinus rhythm if it occurs after myocardial infarction or cardiac surgery. Conversion to sinus rhythm is the primary aim of treatment, but this may be difficult to maintain in some patients with longstanding atrial fibrillation. In these patients, the ventricular response to the atria can be controlled with digoxin (*see* p. 106).

Atrial flutter (Fig. 3.31)

Rhythm	regularly irregular
P waves	saw-toothed appearance of base line at about 300 times/minute known as F or flutter waves
QRS	normal

The atrial impulses of about 300 per minute are partially blocked at the AV node. This block is desirable, because if there was 1 : 1 conduction the ventricles would also contract at 300 times per minute, which would produce a totally inadequate cardiac output.

Causes, nursing intervention and treatment are as for atrial fibrillation, but atrial flutter reverts easily at cardioversion with a 25 – 50 joule shock.

Junctional rhythm (Fig. 3.32)

Rhythm	regular
Rate	50 – 70 per minute usually
P waves	none seen
QRS duration	normal

This rhythm looks like sinus rhythm but there are no P waves as impulses originate in the AV junctional tissue, then are conducted to the ventricles in the normal manner, hence the QRS complex will be narrow. Sometimes the impulse may travel from the junction in a retrograde fashion back to the atria, to cause an inverted P wave before, during, or after the QRS complex (Fig. 3.32).

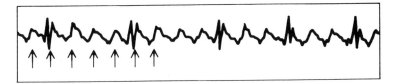

Fig. 3.31 Atrial flutter. F waves are narrowed.

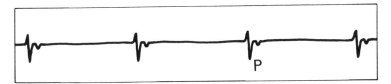

Fig. 3.32 Junctional rhythm with retrograde P wave.

CAUSES

An escape rhythm in the absence of a sinus rhythm. An accelerated ectopic rhythm, commonly following inferior myocardial ischaemia, infarction, or digoxin toxicity.

NURSING INTERVENTION

The patient is usually asymptomatic and no action is necessary, unless the rate is very fast. Document the rhythm in the nursing records and mention to medical staff.

AV dissociation (Fig. 3.33)

Rhythm	regular except for two apparently premature beats
Rate	ventricular rate 71 and faster than the P wave rate of 69
P waves	appear to 'walk through' the QRS complexes
PR interval	varying relationship, but before each 'premature' beat, the preceding T wave appears to have a P wave superimposed on it. These two P waves occur far enough away from the preceding QRS complex and

so find the AV node repolarized and able to pass the atrial impulse to the ventricles in a normal manner. These 'premature' beats are called capture beats

AV dissociation is a combination of an accelerated junctional or ventricular escape rhythm and a slower sinus rhythm which it has overtaken.

Causes, action and treatment are the same as for junctional rhythm, but the rhythm should be differentiated from other types of AV block, and digoxin toxicity closely considered.

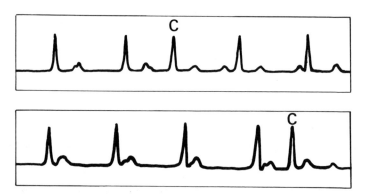

Fig. 3.33   AV dissociation showing capture beats.

Ectopic beats

These may originate in the atria, junction, or ventricles. The shape of the premature QRS complex or P wave, and their relationship to the underlying rhythm, will indicate the site of the ectopic focus (*see* p. 46). The patient will not usually be aware of these ectopic beats but ectopics indicate that the area is irritable and tachycardias or fibrillation could follow.

ATRIAL ECTOPIC BEATS (Fig. 3.34)

RR intervals	regular except the interval before the premature beat is shorter
Rhythm	underlying rhythm is sinus rhythm
P waves	identical except for an abnormal P wave before the premature beat
QRS complexes	normal, including the premature beat

Causes
As for atrial fibrillation

Nursing intervention
None necessary as the patient would be asymptomatic, but if the ectopics are frequent they could lead to atrial fibrillation.

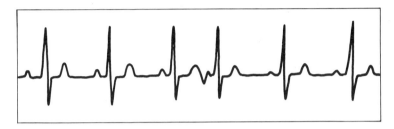

Fig. 3.34 Atrial ectopic beat

JUNCTIONAL ECTOPIC BEATS   *no P*

Rhythm   very similar to Fig. 3.34 but there would be no P waves
             before the premature beats

As with junctional rhythms, the ectopic focus is in the AV junction which may conduct an impulse retrogradely to the atria to produce a premature QRS complex with a mishapen P wave before, during, or after it.

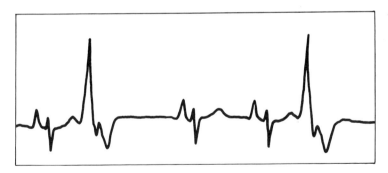

Fig. 3.35 Ventricular ectopic beats.

VENTRICULAR ECTOPIC BEATS (Fig. 3.35)   *no P.   bizarre QRS . T*

The underlying rhythm is sinus with two very noticeable bizarre, wide premature beats. These have no preceding P wave and the T waves are of opposite polarity to the T waves of the sinus beats. In Fig. 3.35 the atria have been activated retrogradely, as shown by the P wave after the ectopic beats.

Pulse
The sinus rhythm would produce a regular pulse, but the ectopic beats would not be felt at all nor would they disturb the underlying rhythm. The pulse will feel as if whole beats are missed.

Causes
These beats may occur in normal hearts after stimulants of caffeine and nicotine. Ventricular irritability from hypoxia, acidosis, hypokalaemia, and catecholamine release in fear, pain and anxiety will cause ventricular ectopics in vulnerable patients (*see* p. 59).

Nursing intervention
Ventricular ectopics indicate that the ventricles are irritable, in a vulnerable patient these ectopics are warnings that ventricular tachycardia or fibrillation could occur any second. Action to treat or suppress the irritable ventricles is indicated if:
1 There are frequent ventricular ectopics (more than six per minute).
2 There are multifocal ectopics (i.e. the ectopics are of different shapes indicating that there is more than one ectopic focus within the ventricles) (Fig. 3.36).
3 Ectopics fall on the T wave of the preceding beat (*see* R on T phenomenon p. 59).
4 There are salvos of ectopic beats (i.e. two or more ectopics occur together)(Fig. 3.37).

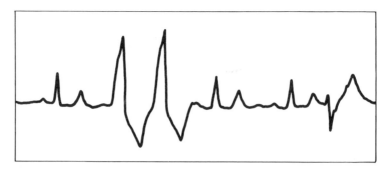

Fig. 3.36 Multifocal ventricular ectopic beats.

Record a rhythm tracing, but do not alarm the patient. Relieve any pain or anxiety if possible and call a doctor. In many coronary units, the doctor will have inserted an i.v. cannula when the patient was admitted with a suspected myocardial infarction. Intravenous drugs may have been prescribed in anticipation of ventricular ectopics (or severe bradycardias). It is the nurse who observes the monitor and diagnoses the rhythm, the nurse then gives the drugs at her discretion to prevent life-threatening arrhythmias developing, e.g. ventricular tachycardia or fibrillation.

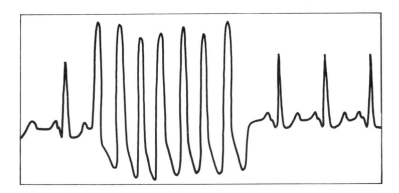

Fig. 3.37 A salvo of ventricular tachycardia.

Treatment

None if the ectopics are isolated, but consider if the patient has a reason to have an irritable myocardium and treat any hypoxia, acidosis, or hypokalaemia. If the patient is receiving any inotropic agents, such as adrenaline, consider if these can be reduced.

Administer anti-arrhythmic drugs, e.g. i.v. lignocaine 50 – 100 mg bolus followed by an infusion of lignocaine at a rate of 2 – 4 mg per minute. Lignocaine lasts only a short time in the body so, if the infusion is stopped, the effect will stop within 15 minutes. Lignocaine suppresses the irritable ventricle, but is only slightly negatively inotropic. At an infusion rate of more than 4 mg/minute the patient may hallucinate, fit, or stop breathing. Lignocaine has no effect on supra-ventricular ectopics and cannot be given orally. Other drugs that may be considered include disopyramide (i.v. bolus slowly, infusion then orally), mexiletine (i.v. bolus slowly, infusion then orally), bretylium (i.v. bolus slowly and repeat), beta blocking agents, practolol (i.v. bolus slowly), propranolol (i.v. bolus slowly, then orally).

Differential diagnosis

The nurse must be able to differentiate between potentially harmful ventricular ectopics that require treatment, and supraventricular ectopics that do not. There are three main distinguishing features. **1** Ventricular ectopics are usually bizarre and wide, whereas the QRS complex of a supraventricular ectopic is narrow and will look identical or very similar to the QRS complexes of the underlying rhythm. **2** In addition, the T wave following a ventricular ectopic will usually be opposite in polarity and bizarre compared to the T waves of the underlying rhythm. Following a supraventricular ectopic, the T wave will usually be unchanged, however T wave inversion can occur after the QRS following the premature beat. **3** Finally, following a supraventricular ectopic (Fig. 3.38), there may appear to be a pause but, when the RR intervals are measured out, the pause will probably be an optical illusion. Following a ventricular ectopic (Fig. 3.39) there is a pause, said to be fully compensatory because the sinus node waits to depolarize at its preset time, so the underlying rhythm is not disturbed.

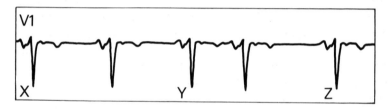

Fig. 3.38 Sinus rhythm with a supraventricular ectopic beat (the 4th P wave). The post ectopic pause is incomplete as ascertained by measuring the RR intervals, distance YZ is less than distance XY.

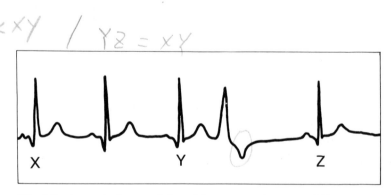

Fig. 3.9 A ventricular ectopic beat. The post ectopic pause is fully compensatory as ascertained by distance XY being equal to distance YZ.

Ventricular tachycardia (Fig. 3.40)

Rhythm	slightly irregular
P waves	cannot be clearly identified
Rate	may be 80 – 300 per minute
QRS duration	prolonged

CAUSES

Ventricular irritability in susceptible patients, e.g. myocardial ischaemia or infarction. Repeated episodes of this tachycardia can be caused by a ventricular aneurysm, or scar of a myocardial infarction.

NURSING INTERVENTION

Without alarming the patient by your actions, rapidly assess his general condition; some patients may be only slightly disturbed by this dangerous rhythm, others will be shocked. Call the medical staff immediately, record a monitor rhythm tracing. Next, prepare (and administer if unit policy allows) i.v. lignocaine, and then prepare other anti-arrhythmics and the defibrillator, as ventricular fibrillation frequently follows ventricular tachycardia. Treat the cause if possible, e.g. hypoxia, pain, or hypokalaemia. Recurring tachycardia may be terminated by overpacing, or investigations and surgery may be indicated for a few patients who are not immediately post-infarction or post-surgery.

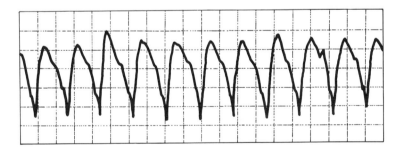

Fig. 3.40   Ventricular tachycardia.

Ventricular fibrillation (Fig. 3.41)

In this figure, the first four beats are sinus rhythm (with evidence of a recent inferior myocardial infarction), the fifth beat is a ventricular ectopic that falls on the T wave of the preceding beat, R on T, and the rhythm is then disorganized in shape, size and rate, no clear PQRST complexes can be identified.

CAUSES

These include extreme ventricular irritability, e.g. post-infarction or cardiac surgery.

NURSING INTERVENTION

Cardiac output will cease. The patient will become unconscious, the pulse will stop, pupils will dilate and respirations will be gasping and then stop. A short hypoxic fit may occur. Commence the cardiac arrest procedure (*see* p. 140). Defibrillate the patient with 200 – 400 joules immediately. After conversion, give anti-arrhythmic drugs to prevent recurrence.

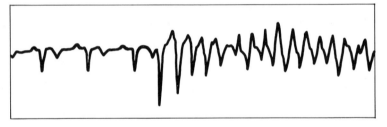

Fig. 3.41   Ventricular fibrillation.

Heart block

Disease of the specialized conducting tissues within the heart gives a number of clearly recognizable patterns on the ECG or cardiac monitor for the nurse to observe, diagnose, and initiate appropriate treatment.

ATRIOVENTRICULAR NODE BLOCK

Impulses originating in the sinus node or atrium can be blocked or delayed at the AV junction. Depending on the severity of the block this may result in: prolonged PR intervals, P waves occasionally not followed by QRS complexes, or P waves never followed by QRS complexes. Fortunately the bundle of His or ventricles will usually supply a slower escape rhythm, should the P waves all be blocked. The escape rhythms originating in the ventricles will be much slower than the sinus rate and very unreliable; in addition the QRS complexes will be wide and bizarre.

Causes of AV block

1 Fibrosis of the conducting tissue with age.

2 Transient ischaemia of the AV node following myocardial infarction (commonly inferior infarction). Heart block only follows anterior myocardial infarction if the infarction is extensive; heart block in these patients is therefore a bad prognostic sign.

3 Calcification of the aortic valve which is involving the bundle of His.

4 Congenital heart block.

5 Transient oedema following surgery to the septum or aortic valve.

6 Drugs that slow AV conduction: digoxin, beta blockers, disopyramide, quinidine.

7 Myocarditis.

8 Ankylosing spondylitis.

The patient's symptoms will vary according to how much the cardiac output is dependent on the rate, and how severe the underlying myocardial disease is. Some patients experience syncope and Stokes-Adams attacks when a slow heart rate drops the cardiac output dramatically, or if the heart action and cardiac output cease altogether for several seconds. A constantly slow heart rate in patients who have compromised myocardial function, e.g. after myocardial infarction or surgery, may develop heart failure and shock. Patients with more normal myocardial function will develop chronic heart failure over a period of weeks or months.

[margin handwriting: normal breath 30 sec, pale, attach, flush, hot, awake]

Nursing intervention

The ventricular rate will usually determine what action is necessary. Assess the patient's apex beat, respiration, blood pressure, skin temperature and mental alertness. Record a monitor rhythm tracing. Depending on assessment no action may be immediately necessary apart from recording in the nursing records and informing the medical staff later. If the patient's cardiac output is seriously compromised, or heart action has ceased altogether, then the cardiac arrest procedure should be instituted.

Treatment

Treatment will also vary according to the degree of block and the patient's symptoms. Drugs can be given that increase AV conduction. Atropine 0.6 – 1.2 mg is the first drug of choice for bradycardia and heart block. This has a chronotropic effect only. Adrenaline and isoprenaline increase AV conduction with their chronotropic effect, but they also increase myocardial contractility and irritability. These effects are desirable in complete block as they will stimulate ventricular escape rhythms. Temporary or permanent pacing may be commenced.

Drugs that are known to impair AV conduction will be reduced or discontinued. Unless the patient has a pacemaker inserted, patients with heart block should not be given anti-arrhythmic drugs to suppress ectopic beats, as the potentially life-saving escape rhythms will also be suppressed. A post-cardiac surgery oedema may cause heart block and intravenous hydrocortisone may be effective.

FIRST DEGREE AV BLOCK (*see* Fig. 3.3)

PR interval	lengthened over 0.2 seconds
QRS complexes	narrow
	each P wave is followed by a QRS complex

The patient would be unaffected by this partial block so no immediate action is necessary. Record a rhythm tracing and document in the nursing records. This block may progress to a more serious block post-infarction or surgery and will need close observation.

SECOND DEGREE AV BLOCK

There are two types of this partial block.

Mobitz type 1 (Wenckebach) (Fig. 3.42)   *PR intervals* ⟶
This may follow first degree block, and indicates that the AV node or bundle of His is having more and more difficulty conducting, e.g. due to ischaemia. It is quite common after inferior myocardial infarction. PR intervals progressively lengthen until a QRS complex is dropped allowing the junction to recover and the cycle is repeated. The PQRST complexes appear to group together. The QRS complexes are narrow and normal looking. The RR intervals become progressively shorter before the missed QRS complex.

The patient will not usually be aware of this change in rhythm, and nursing action is the same as for first degree block. It is unlikely that the patient will develop complete heart block but the doctor should be notified and the patient closely observed.

Mobitz type 2 (Fig. 3.43)

PR interval	constant (unlike Wenckebach or complete block)
QRS complex	normal and narrow usually
P waves	more P waves than QRS complexes but they may be buried in preceding T wave

This indicates a more serious partial block in the AV junction and could lead on to complete heart block. It may randomly stop conduction of P waves or a regular partial block may develop that blocks altenate P waves: two out of three P waves or three out of four waves. (In atrial tachyarrhythmias, a partial block of this type is desirable, e.g. if the atria flutter at 300, a 2 : 1 AV block will produce a ventricular rate of 150/minute.)

The patient may be unaware of the change in rhythm, or he may become profoundly shocked. This will depend on the ventricular rate and the patient's underlying myocardial disease.

Nursing intervention
Assess the patient's general condition, and record a monitor rhythm tracing. Then inform the medical staff, giving all relevant information of ventricular rate and general condition. Finally, observe the patient closely and prepare intravenous atropine.

Second degree block may be a chronic and stable rhythm in elderly patients, but chronic heart failure may be precipitated. This should respond to diuretics. Permanent pacing will be considered if the ventricular rate is low, and diuretic therapy alone is ineffective in these patients. Acute onset of heart block often occurs after inferior myocardial infarction, and usually lasts a few days or up to two weeks.

Intravenous atropine, isoprenaline infusion or temporary pacing may be used if the patient is symptomatic.

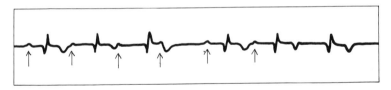

Fig. 3.42   Second degree AV (Wenckebach) block. P waves are arrowed.

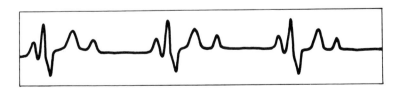

Fig. 3.43   Second degree (Mobitz type II) block.

THIRD DEGREE BLOCK (Fig. 3.44)

P waves	more frequent than QRS complexes
PR interval	varies before each QRS
P wave – QRS	P waves have no relationship to QRS complexes

In the acute infarction or post-surgical patients, this heart block may progress on from second degree block. Complete heart block may be due to blockage of the AV node, bundles of His, or if all fascicles of the bundle branches are blocked (*see* p. 56).

Episodes of complete block may occur without a reliable escape rhythm in otherwise healthy elderly individuals to cause Stokes – Adams attacks.

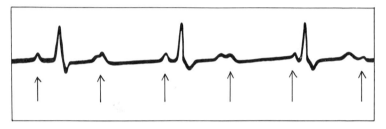

Fig. 3.44   Complete third degree block.

STOKES – ADAMS ATTACKS

These are periods of low or no cardiac output that cause the patient to feel faint, dizzy and fall to the ground unconscious. The patient becomes deathly white and pulseless due to cessation of all cardiac output. What distinguishes a Stokes – Adams attack from certain death is that the block is only transient, or an escape rhythm takes over to return heart action and cardiac output. When cardiac output is restored, the patient will flush pink and regain consciousness. Repeated attacks may cause cerebral hypoxia and brain damage.

Heart block case study

An 85-year-old lady was admitted to hospital with a history of dizzy spells and episodes of loss of consciousness which caused her to fall to the ground. Apart from these episodes she was a fit lady who cared for herself and her husband in their own home. She was mentally fully alert but, since the dizzy spells had begun, she had become housebound because of the fear of fainting in the street. She had suffered several attacks the previous day, so her husband had called the doctor who examined her and arranged an ambulance to take her to hospital. Her ECG showed sinus rhythm with a bundle branch block pattern. Her blood pressure, temperature and respirations were normal. No neurological deficit could be found to account for her dizzy spells.

Because of her history of repeated syncopal attacks and the bundle branch block on her ECG, she was attached to a cardiac monitor for observation and an intravenous cannula was inserted; later that day the tracing shown in Fig. 3.45 was taken.

Note the complete AV block with a slow ventricular escape rhythm, and that a period of ventricular standstill occurred when the unreliable escape rhythm stopped. The patient became dizzy, then unconscious and pulseless but fortunately the escape rhythm returned and she flushed pink and regained her pulse and consciousness. The doctor was notified and an infusion of isoprenaline 5 mg in 500 ml was commenced at 40 ml per hour.

The diagnosis was explained to the patient and her husband and an immediate temporary, then a permanent, pacemaker was advised.

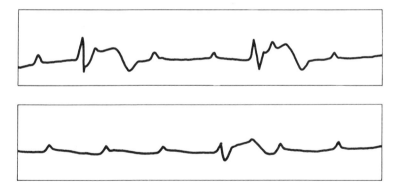

Fig. 3.45 Complete heart block (*above*) leading to (*below*) a Stokes–Adams attack.

SINOATRIAL NODE DISEASE

The sinus node initiates the P wave of atrial depolarization. The diseased sinus node may fail altogether, be blocked, or initiate too many P waves at irregular intervals. Sinus node depolarization itself does not produce any waves on the ECG, but a pre P wave stimulus can be imagined.

Sinus Wenckebach

The sinus impulse will be progressively delayed leaving the node, until one impulse is blocked altogether. The RR intervals will shorten, then there will be one longer RR interval causing a pause, and then the cycle is repeated.

Second degree sinus block (Fig. 3.46)

Unlike sinus Wenckebach, the RR intervals will remain constant, until one whole PQRST complex is dropped.

Sinus arrest

In sinus arrest, the impulse will fail to leave the sinus node. No P waves or QRS complexes will be seen and asystole will follow, unless a junctional or ventricular escape rhythm is established.

Wandering atrial pacemaker

The P waves will be of different shapes and sizes, the RR and PR intervals will also be different due to impulses arising from different parts of the atrium and occasionally from the sinus node.

The patient will be unaware of most of the above rhythm disturbances, but may feel dizzy or lose consciousness during sinus arrest pauses.

Causes

These include uraemia, ischaemia, myocarditis, drugs or can be idiopathic.

Nursing intervention and treatment are the same as for AV block.

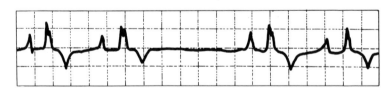

Fig. 3.46 Second degree sinus block.

ARRHYTHMIAS AND PACING

Fast arrhythmias

TACHYBRADYCARDIA

This is a disturbance of normal rhythm, with bouts of tachycardia up to 180/minute then extreme bradycardia down to or less than 40/minute. The causes are as for an AV block. The patient will experience palpitations, dizziness, and possible syncope with a change in skin colour from pale to flushed as cardiac output drops, then returns to normal. This is very distressing for the patient.

Treatment
Treatment is difficult because drugs to slow the tachycardia will increase the bradycardic episodes. Permanent pacing to prevent the bradycardias will allow treatment of the tachycardias with drugs such as beta blockers, verapamil or disopyramide. Surgical division of the tachycardia focus may be carried out if the arrhythmia is resistant to pacing and drugs. His bundle studies and cardiac mapping will be carried out and the irritant focus excised or the pathway divided at open heart surgery.

TACHYCARDIAS

Recurrent tachycardias that are resistant to drugs can sometimes be terminated with overpacing — a few paced beats at 200 – 400/minute act like cardioversion to capture all the atrial and ventricular muscle, causing simultaneous depolarization. The sinus node is usually the most rapidly repolarizing tissue, a sinus rhythm can therefore be restored without the trauma of repeated cardioversion.

A temporary transvenous pacemaker is inserted and it can be controlled by an experienced nurse once its effectiveness has been proved. Special permanent pacing systems can be built for patients with paroxysmal life-threatening tachycardias that are resistant to other treatments.

Slow arrhythmias

If the patient has a slow or potentially slow heart rate, with symptoms of dizziness, syncope, or heart failure, these can be treated by raising the rate with drugs such as atropine, adrenaline, or isoprenaline. These drugs can be effective for a few hours or days in most patients but they have undesirable side-effects. A more reliable method, which can be temporary or permanent, is regular electrical stimulation of the myocardium by an electrode attached to a battery and pulse generator.

A fixed pacemaker is one that sends out impulses to the myocardium at a regular and constant rate, whether the heart requires a pacing stimulus or not. However, most patients, even in complete block, have occasional beats of their own, and if a pacing impulse were to fall on the T wave of the preceding beat (R on T phenomenon), ventricular fibrillation could occur. Fixed pacemakers are rarely fitted for this reason.

Demand pacemakers avoid the R on T phenomenon because they have an inbuilt mechanism which can *sense* when the patient has a QRS complex and which *inhibits* the pacemaker from sending an impulse. The pacemaker is then said to be 'on demand', i.e. it will fire only when it is required.

A permanent pacemaker is usually set at a demand rate of 70 in an adult. The rate of temporary pacemakers can be set at almost any rate.

Pacing and the ECG

The electrical stimulus from the pacemaker can be seen on the ECG as a spike preceding the QRS complex (Fig. 3.47). If the stimulus has caused myocardial stimulation, that is if it has 'captured' the ventricles, the spike will be immediately followed by a wide ventricular QRS complex and a pulse can be felt. If it does not capture the ventricules, the ECG will show a spike but no QRS and no pulse will be felt.

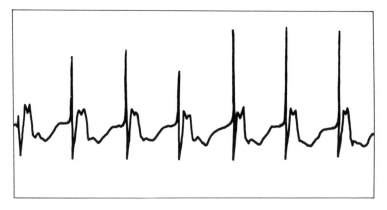

Fig. 3.47 Continuous pacing.

Good demand pacing (Fig. 3.48)

The patient's own rhythm has narrow QRS complexes. A large pacing spike is followed by a wide QRS complex when the patient's own rate slows. The last paced beat looks different to the other four, it has fused with a QRS complex initiated by the patient as the underlying rhythm speeds up. It is therefore called a *fusion beat*.

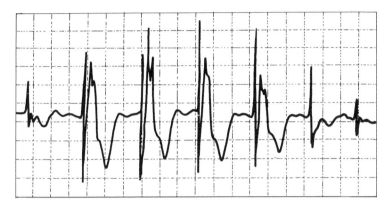

Fig. 3.48 Good demand pacing with a fusion beat.

Failure to capture

Fig. 3.49 shows intermittent failure to capture. Note pacing spikes but no QRS.

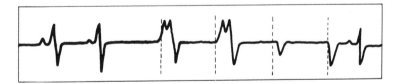

Fig. 3.49 Intermittent failure to capture by pacemaker.

ATRIAL PACING

Atrial pacemakers are inserted when the sinus node is diseased but the AV node is conducting normally. This retains the pause between atrial and ventricular contraction.

Similarly, *synchronous atrial and ventricular pacing* is used for some patients with AV block if atrial contraction is considered essential to maintain cardiac output. Up to 30% of the cardiac output is lost if synchronized atrial contraction is absent (Fig. 3.50).

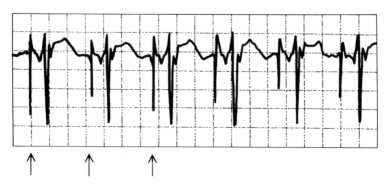

Fig. 3.50 Atrial pacing.

Rhythm	regular
Pacing spike	0.2 seconds before each QRS (arrowed)
P wave	inverted after each pacing spike
QRS	narrrow

Batteries
Mercury cell batteries last reliably for 4 – 5 years. Nuclear batteries last much longer, but they are much more expensive. One barrier to improved battery life is that the battery must be small and light enough to implant in the body. A heavy pacing system would cause discomfort and increase the likelihood of tissue dragging and skin breakdown, both of which predispose to infection.

The pacing wire
The pacing wire needs a positive and a negative pole. A bipolar wire has the two poles near the tip. The impulse passes from one pole to the other so activating the myocardium. A unipolar wire, with one pole at the tip, needs the metal case of an implanted pacemaker or a wire skin stitch to act as the negative pole.

For the myocardium to receive the small electrical pulse from the pacemaker, the wire must be positioned either within the myocardium or very close to it. An *endocardial* wire will be passed via a large vein (using X-ray control) until it reaches the apex of the right ventricle where it will lodge in the trabeculae (Fig. 3.51, a or b). This wire can be attached to an internal or external pacemaker. The technique is described in detail below. An *epicardial* wire will be screwed or stitched into the epicardial surface of the heart at operation. It will be attached to an internal pacemaker (Fig. 3.51 c). This technique is described on p. 90. *Transthoracic* wires may be inserted directly into the heart through the chest wall, either as an emergency procedure using a trocar, or during open heart surgery for use in the immediate post-operative period.

Insertion of a transvenous endocardial pacing wire

One large group of patients with heart block who require permanent pacemakers will be otherwise healthy 80 – 90-year-old people. Other patients with heart block or bradycardias from a number of causes (including post-myocardial infarction) may require only temporary pacing. Some patients may have recurrent tachycardias that can be reverted by overpacing.

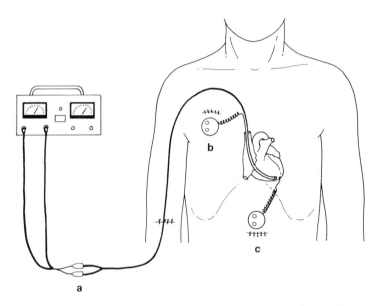

Fig. 3.51 Positioning of transvenous and epicardial pacemakers. **a** Temporary transvenous endocardial pacing wire in the apex of the right ventricle connected to a portable pacemaker box. Here shown inserted in the antecubital fossa but the subclavian or jugular veins could be used instead.
b Permanent pacing system embedded in the pectoral muscle and attached to an endocardial wire.
c Epicardial pacing system in which the wire is screwed into the myocardium and attached to a permanent pacemaker in the abdomen.

POSSIBLE COMPLICATIONS DURING INSERTION

Cardiac arrest.
Inhalation of vomit.
Infection at site of insertion, septicaemia or bacterial endocarditis on any

heart defect or damaged valve.

Patient anxiety and discomfort.

Difficulty in finding a suitable vein to insert the wire.

Difficulty in stabilizing the wire with a low threshold.

Perforation of the ventricle resulting in tamponade.

To minimize these risks the patient should be adequately prepared, and the procedure should be carried out under X-ray control. Occasionally insertion is carried out as an emergency on the ward without fluoroscopic control. In this case, attach the proximal end of the wire to a 12 lead ECG chest lead; this will indicate when the atrium and ventricle have been entered by the change in P wave and QRS shape.

PATIENT PREPARATION

In most cases, in spite of the urgency of inserting the pacemaker wire, there will be time for the doctor fully to explain to the patient why pacing is needed and what the procedure will entail. A written consent form should be obtained unless the procedure is carried out as an extreme emergency. Further explanations from the nurse are usually necessary and should be readily given in a reassuring manner.

The patient will be fasted, to minimise the risk of vomiting and inhaling in the event of cardiac arrest. Other theatre preparations should include the wearing of a cotton gown, removal of metal objects, false teeth, etc; however, if the patient normally wears a hearing aid, this should not be removed so the patient can listen to explanations and answer questions during the procedure.

If possible, the patient's haemoglobin and electrolytes should be checked and should be within normal limits prior to the procedure.

The expected site of insertion should be shaved and cleaned. The medial antecubital or subclavian vein is commonly used for inserting a temporary pacing wire, while a permanent wire is often placed through the internal jugular vein.

A premedication of papaveretum or diazepam may be given, but it is usually safer to give small intravenous doses of sedatives or opiates during the procedure, depending on the patient's general condition. The procedure is carried out using local anaesthetic, so explanations and reassurance by the ward and X-ray nurse are essential.

PROCEDURE

Insertion of an endocardial pacing wire will be carried out in the angiography department, the X-ray department, or the coronary care unit if it has a portable image intensifier. Full rescusitation equipment should be ready for use.

The patient is attached to ECG monitoring and an i.v. cannula is inserted. Under local anaesthetic and using an aseptic technique, a cut down or direct vein puncture is performed and the pacing wire is then advanced along the vein towards the heart. Using X-ray control, the wire is manipulated into the right atrium, through the tricuspid valve and into the apex of the right ventricle. The passage of the wire may cause ventricular tachycardia or fibrillation, but once it is lodged in the trabeculae at the apex, the wire should not cause irritation of the ventricle or move on coughing or other movement.

Next the wire is then attached to an external pacing box and its *threshold* is checked. The threshold is the smallest voltage needed to stimulate (capture) the ventricles to produce a QRS complex reliably. If the wire is in a good position, the threshold should be 1.0 volt or less. The threshold on temporary systems should be checked daily and recorded. This involves reducing the voltage set on the box slowly while observing the monitor or feeling the pulse. When below-threshold is reached, failure to capture will result in a spike on the ECG but no QRS complex or pulse (*see* Fig. 3.49). The voltage should then be turned up immediately and set at 1.5 – 2 times the threshold as a safety margin. An unnecessarily high voltage could result in ventricular arrthymias. Similarly, if failure to capture is noted at any other time, the nurse should increase the voltage on the box and then notify the medical staff.

If pacing is only a temporary measure, the wire will be attached to an external pacing system. The pulse generator and battery box will be attached to the pacing wire by a lead and junction box or clips. The wire will be securely sutured and strapped in position. If pacing is to be permanent, a small sealed pulse generator and battery box will be attached to the wire, then put in a pouch made in the patient's pectoral muscle. The pouch is then sutured closed; a drain is not usually necessary, but a pressure dressing will be applied.

POSSIBLE COMPLICATIONS AFTER INSERTION

Haemorrhage or haematoma at insertion site (or box pouch).
Pneumothorax if the subclavian approach has been used.
Displacement of the wire. Perforation of the wire through the right ventricle — possibly causing tamponade.
Arrythymias caused by irritation of the wire in the ventricle. Irritation is marked if the wire accidently lies in the pulmonary artery outflow tract.
Infections — septicaemia or local wound infections.
Patient discomfort and restriction.

The patient should be closely observed on return to the ward in case these complications develop. Respiration, pulse, blood pressue, wound site and the patient's general condition should be observed closely at 15 minute intervals initially. The patient should be connected to a cardiac monitor to check for signs of wire displacement and arrhythmias (*see* Fig. 3.49).

Any problems usually occur within one or two days of insertion, though at any time a wire may crack or become displaced due to blunt injury or a sudden body movement such as tripping over. A *cracked wire* causes total or intermittent failure to pace, as shown by the lack of pacing spikes on the ECG during this time. If no escape rhythm occurs, ventricular standstill will result and the patient will die or experience Stokes – Adams attacks. A *displaced wire* will move away from the endocardium, either to float within the heart or to perforate the myocardium, thus causing pericarditis or possibly pacing the diaphragm, which would be very painful. With wire displacement, pacing spikes appear on the ECG but they continually or intermittently fail to capture (Fig. 3.49).

Unreliable pacing, with failure to sense and inhibit and/or failure to capture, may be due to oedema occurring in the tissues around the tip of the wire. Steroids may help. Pacing will also be unreliable if the tip of the wire is against an ischaemic or fibrosed part of the myocardium.

Unsatisfactory wire positioning will cause the threshold on the wire to rise. A chest X-ray will show any shift in wire position which should be corrected under theatre conditions, as for insertion.

To minimise the risk of wire displacement or perforation, some centres discourage the patient from lying on their right side for 24 hours after insertion; also if the antecubital approach has been used for a temporary wire, the arm may be immobilized. Unless the wire is known to be unstable, these measures are not usually necessary and the patient can immediately sit up in bed if he wishes. The next day, if the patient's general condition allows, he should be encouraged to be fully mobile and independent. If the pacemaker is a temporary one, the patient should be shown how to carry his pacing box safely. The nurse should ensure that the wires and junction box are secure and do not drag. The wire terminals should be prevented from touching each other, or the paced impulse could short across these terminals instead of stimulating the heart and asystole could occur.

Since the wire is in contact with the myocardium, extra care is needed not to expose the patient to potentially hazardous electrical equipment, such as ECG machines or electrical razors. Ventricular fibrillation can occur if even a small voltage accidently passes down the wire. In addition patients who have demand pacemakers should be warned that these may be falsely inhibited by radiation from infra-red ovens.

Prophylactic antibiotics are usually prescribed while the temporary wire is in situ. The wound should be inspected and a dry dressing applied aseptically each day. Wound inflammation, excessive pain, or pyrexia will indicate an infection is present.

Some pain, and certainly discomfort, will be felt by the patient who has had a permanent pacemaker implanted. Oral or intramuscular dihydrocodeine may be needed for the first day, but paracetamol should be sufficient later. If excessive pain is experienced, this indicates infection or a haematoma in the pouch. Normally the discomfort and swelling over the implanted box should subside after 1 – 2 weeks, leaving a small bulge under the skin. This bulge will be more noticeable in slim individuals, who should take extra care not to knock or damage the skin over the box.

Removal of a temporary transvenous wire

The temporary wire can be removed when pacing is no longer necessary, or a permanent system has been inserted and checked. Before the wire is removed the patient must be reassured that he no longer needs the wire; some patients become psychologically dependent on their pacing boxes.

PROCEDURE

The patient should be resting in or on the bed. If the pacemaker has been left turned to 'on demand' it should be turned off prior to its removal, otherwise the pacing impulse will cause painful and disturbing muscle twitching when the wire is pulled out of the heart.

Using an aseptic technique, remove the sutures that are holding the wire in place and clean the wound. To detect any ventricular arrhythmias that could occur as the wire is pulled out throught the heart, observe the monitor or feel the patient's pulse. Remove the wire with a slow and gentle pulling motion so that it will not flick the ventricular walls or tricuspid valve to cause arrhythmias. Apply a small dry dressing for a day or two. Wash the wire in soap and water and return it to the cardiac department for possible re-use.

Transthoracic pacing wires inserted during an open heart procedure are removed by a gentle pulling motion when they are no longer needed — about the third post-operative day. When in situ, the wires should be secured with tape and individually labelled: 'ventricular', 'atrial' or 'indifferent'.

Insertion of an epicardial pacing wire

A wire is either sewn or screwed into the outside of the heart wall and the pulse generator and battery are embedded behind the rectus sheath in the abdomen.

Epicardial pacing systems are inserted:

1 When it is impossible to maintain a good threshold on an endocardial wire, e.g. in dilated or fibrosed hearts.
2 In children because an endocardial transvenous wire would become displaced by growth.
3 To reduce the risk of endocarditis in patients with valve disease or other intracardiac abnormalities.
4 To implant the box in a totally different area in patients who have repeated infections at the box insertion site.

All patients will need to have a transvenous temporary wire in situ in case heart block is aggrevated by induction of anaesthesia.

POSSIBLE COMPLICATIONS

Following the operation, the patient should be observed for the same complications as for the endocardial pacing wire; however, wire displacement is rare. In addition it must be remembered that these patients are often elderly and they have undergone a modified thorocotomy and general anaesthetic. They will require more analgesia, chest physiotherapy, and slower post-operative mobilization.

Pacemaker checking

The function of the pacemaker and wire will be checked before the patient goes home. Also a PA and left lateral chest X-ray will be taken to see the position of the wire and box. A technician will record an ECG tracing and calculate the rate and height of the pacing impulses. Demand pacemakers have an inbuilt facility to switch to a fixed mode by placing a magnet over the box. This will enable checking of the pacemaker impulses, even when the patient's own rate is faster than the demand mode.

Repeat checking of the pacemaker will be done after a month and then once a year. When the batteries are nearing the end of their expected life, it will be checked more frequently. Arrangements for changing the pacing box will be made when the batteries are seen to be running down.

Urgent admission and insertion of a temporary pacing system will be necessary if the generator, battery, wire, or wire position are faulty. Patients may experience recurrent Stokes–Adams attacks or acute heart failure if their pacing system suddenly fails.

CHANGING THE PACING SYSTEM

A general anaesthetic will be necesary to remove the old box as it will be surrounded by tissue adhesions. A temporary wire will need to be inserted first if the old system is faulty, but if it is just running low, there is no risk of asystole at induction of the anaesthetic. The wire will be inspected and its threshold checked; if this is unacceptably high or faulty, then it too will be changed.

AFTERCARE

Patients with a permanent endocardial system will usually be mobilized, have their pacemakers checked, and be ready for discharge by the second or third post-operative day. An elderly patient may need to stay with relatives for a few days, but most patients can go straight home. The district nurse may need to be contacted to remove any silk sutures in 7 – 10 days, or younger fitter patients could visit their general practitioner for this. Following the operation to implant an epicardial system, the patient will be mobilized more slowly, and ready for discharge in 6 – 7 days.

Teaching the patient or a relative to feel the pulse may be helpful to detect abnormalities but there are problems. Any discrepancy in the pulse may be due to ectopics or atrial fibrillation and not to pacing failure, thus the patient could be unduly alarmed and constantly worry about his pulse without good reason. The nurse should therefore use her discretion before showing every patient how to take their pulse.

The fact that a patient has a pacemaker does not mean that they are an invalid. This should be stressed to parents and to relatives of elderly patients who may otherwise place restrictions on the patient's life which will negate the purpose for which the pacemaker was implanted! A full and active life can include full-time work, sports, swimming, air travel, and (if the licencing authorities are informed) car driving — though not bus or lorry driving.

Any problems concerning the pacemaker or other aspects of health should be referred initially to the patient's general practitioner. He will refer the patient to the pacing clinic or hospital if necessary.

Chapter 4
The diseased heart

Heart failure can occur in spite of various compensatory mechanisms to maintain cardiac output. The heart is a muscular pump that should be able to eject a suitable volume of blood against the pressure of the arterial system to satisfy the demands of the tissues.

Heart disease may cause:

1 The muscle pump to beweakened by myocardial disease.

2 An increased *workload* which will impair heart function either by increasing the *volume* of the preload, or the *pressure* of the afterload.

3 Restriction to the filling of the heart chambers.

4 Other diseases may demand a higher cardiac output than even a healthy heart can produce.

CAUSES OF HEART FAILURE

Myocardial dysfunction

This may be caused by: ischaemia or infarction, infections, myocarditis, cardiomyopathy, ventricular aneursym, surgical trauma, hypoxia, acidosis, or electrolyte imbalance. Direct disease of the myocardium will obviously reduce its pumping efficiency. When all the venous return can no longer be ejected into the arteries, cardiac output will fall and the heart chambers will become engorged with blood.

In the presence of a lowered cardiac output, bloodflow to the kidneys will be reduced (*see* p. 37). Sodium and then water will be retained in an effort to increase circulating blood volume. This increase in blood volume returning to the heart will initially improve contractility and cardiac output by Starling's Law (p. 34) and the heart muscle will become thicker (hypertrophy) in an effort to maintain the larger stroke volume. This compensatory mechanism may be effective for many years without any other signs of heart strain occurring.

HYPERTROPHY

Several undesirable effects may occur with hypertrophy which will impair cardiac function.

1 The raised pressure on the stretched ventricle wall will compress the coronary arterioles that nourish the wall, causing ischaemia, angina and infarction. **2** The enlarged muscle will demand more oxygen from the coronary arteries. Ischaemia, angina and infarction may occur. **3** The change in ventricular wall shape may distort the valve rings making them incompetent, so increasing heart failure. **4** The dilated ventricle will allow stasis of blood so thromboli are likely to develop at areas of infarcted, infected, or aneursymal tissue.

Contractility can be improved in the short term by an increase in sympathetic stimulation. This improves the stretch and recoil properties of the muscle fibres and so increases stroke volume. If contractility cannot be improved, then the heart rate will rise to maintain cardiac output.

$$\text{Cardiac output} = \text{rate} \times \text{stroke volume}$$

A persistent sinus tachycardia during recovery from a myocardial infarction or myocarditis for example is a sign that the heart is on the verge of failure. If no excess demands are made upon the heart and the patient is rested, then no further signs of failure may occur.

Low cardiac output may occur earlier in those who are unable to increase their heart rates should their contractility fail, e.g. patients with heart block or abnormally slow heart rates due to sympathetic blocking drugs.

Increased ventricular workload

VOLUME (OR PRELOAD)

This may be caused by mitral or aortic insufficiency, septal defect or patent ductus, and on hearts with borderline reserve with i.v. fluid overload or peritoneal dialysis, oliguric renal failure, or pregnancy.

If heart valves become incompetent or congenital defects of the septum or a patent ductus exist, blood will be ejected by the ventricles in the usual manner, but only a proportion of the cardiac output will be circulated to the tissues. The remainder will be returned via the leaky valves to the ventricles, or with septal defects the blood will pass into the right heart and be re-circulated via the lungs before reaching the left ventricle again. This will result in an increased load on the heart chambers which will hypertrophy and dilate to enable them to eject the larger initial stroke volume needed to ensure adequate blood flow to the tissues. The hypertrophy and dilation will often be effective in children or adults for many years until increased demands are made on the diseased heart by growth, illness, or pregnancy.

PRESSURE (OR AFTERLOAD)

On the left ventricle this may be caused by systemic hypertension, aortic valve stenosis, or coarctation of the aorta. On the right heart, causes are pulmonary disease and pulmonary valve stenosis.

In health, the heart valves offer little resistance to blood flowing in the desired direction, similarly the elastic aorta and arteries will stretch to accommodate the blood ejected at systole. Should the valves become stenosed, or the arteries rigid or constricted by arteriosclerosis or hypertension, the heart will have to work harder to eject the same stroke volume against this increased resistance. Ventricular hypertrophy will occur with increase in muscle mass, but not initially cavity size; however, hypertension falsely triggers fluid retention mechanisms which will also increase the volume load on the ventricle (*see* p. 37).

Restriction of chamber filling

Causes here include mitral stenosis, restrictive pericaditis, restrictive cardiomyopathy, and cardiac tamponade (post surgery or with pericardial effusion).

If the whole heart or just the left ventricle is prevented from filling adequately, then venous congestion and low cardiac output will follow. A tachycardia will be the first compensatory sign of severe restriction to filling, followed by signs of reduced cardiac output (*see also* p. 103.)

Abnormal demands (for increased stroke volume)

This is caused by anaemia, thyrotoxicosis, arrhythmias, or any extensive surgery or overwhelming infection (on a heart with borderline reserve).

In health, the heart can increase its cardiac output up to six times to meet body demands of exercise or other stresses; however, excessive demands (e.g. overwhelming septicaemia, severe anaemia or thyrotoxicosis) may exceed the capability of even a healthy heart.

A higher cardiac output is demanded early in pregnancy, which a healthy heart should be able to supply. Very slow heart rates demand large stroke volumes, and very fast heart rates prevent adequate filling and ejection, cardiac output will fall and other signs of cardiac failure will occur in susceptible patients.

Arrhythmias may contribute to or precipitate heart failure and may be caused by coronary artery disease, thyrotoxicosis or myxoedema, digoxin toxicity, mitral valve disease, hypoxia, electrolyte imbalance, catecholamine release in shocked states, and heart failure. Occasionally arrhythmias also occur in patients with normal hearts.

ATRIAL FIBRILLATION

A hypertrophied heart muscle does not conduct the electrical impulses efficiently and therefore becomes irritable. Atrial fibrillation is thus common in patients with raised left atrial pressure, notably from mitral valve disease. The heart rhythm in atrial fibrillation is completely irregular, with no coordinated atrial contraction to empty the atria or to fill the ventricles. Several effects follow:
1   The atrial pressures rise further as they become dilated with blood, giving pulmonary and systemic venous congestion. 2   The non-contracting walls of the atria allow thrombus formation to occur. 3   The ventricles are not adequately primed to full before conraction, so stroke volume falls.
4   The irregular nature of the ventricular contraction does not allow the heart constant filling time during diastole, stroke volumes will therefore vary with each beat. This means that some beats are felt easily at the radial pulse, but those beats that occur after a short filling time do not produce a palpable radial pulse. 5   The accumulation of the above effects of atrial fibrillation will reduce cardiac output by up to 30%.

Signs and symptoms of heart failure

The numerous signs and symptoms of cardiac disease are shown in Fig. 1.1. For ease of understanding, heart failure is sometimes divided into left or right heart failure, however, left heart failure (especially mitral valve disease) commonly progresses to right heart failure.

LOW CARDIAC OUTPUT

The low blood flow to the kidneys will activate the homeostatic mechanisms of the juxtaglomerular apparatus (*see* p. 37). The patient will have pale, cool, sweaty skin, peripheral cyanosis and a rapid heart rate. He may be anxious, restless and even mentally confused. In less severe low output states, the patient may complain of extreme lethargy, depression, cold hands and feet, and intestinal disturbances of anorexia and constipation.

Table 4.1 (pp. 96-8)   Differential diagnosis of chest pains.

Diagnosis and Character of pain	Location and radiation	Precipitated by or cause
Ischaemic myocardium/angina Dull ache (i.e. not sharp or stabbing) to excruciating pain. Tight choking band round chest	Centre and across. Begins in or spreads to neck, back, abdomen, left and right arm (often inner aspect)	Emotion, exertion, heavy meal, cold weather, trauma, operation (low BP)
Pericarditis Sharp, pleuritic	Ant. chest to back, neck or abdomen	Infection, malignancy, post infarction, allergies, etc.
Myocarditis Very similar to ischaemic pain; not as severe		URT infection, rheumatic fever
Chest infection Dull ache or sharp and pleuritic	Located anywhere in chest, often one side	
Hyperventilation Tight feeling across chest	Across whole ant. chest, tingling to arms, toes and fingers	Anxiety, excitement, a tantrum in children, lowering CO_2 level causing tetany and carpopedal spasm (noticed when B P cuff inflated on arm)
Musculoskeletal Sharp pains and localized tenderness. Area can be pinpointed	Anywhere on chest wall	Recent exertion or trauma

Duration or relieved by	Other signs and symptoms	Treatment
Angina — rest in 20 – 30 min, GTN in 2 – 3 min. Infarction — pain lasts hours, narcotics only	Patient may be shocked, pale, dyspnoeic, sweaty. ECG: ST&T wave changes. BP variable; chest X-ray normal or heart enlarged. Heart rate variable, often fast or irregular	Rest; relieve pain and anxiety. Coronary unit. Investigate GTN. Beta blockers
Pain constant, but relieved by leaning forward. Aspirin, indomethocin	ECG: ST, PR interval & T wave changes. Small QRS voltage or normal. CXR large heart. HR fast. Pyrexia	Rest, aspirin, indomethocin, steroids, narcotics for severe pain. Treat cause. Aspirate effusions if very large
Constant, not GTN	ECG: ST + T changes. Pyrexia	Rest symptomatic relief
Constant or intermittent, not GTN. ?change in body position. Local heat	Pyrexia, cough, infected sputum, suspicious CXR. ECG normal. HR fast	Rest antibiotics, physiotherapy
Relieved by slowing respiration, by calming patient or rebreathing CO_2 in paper bag held over face	Anxiety ++ Tachycardia BP normal ECG & CXR normal	examine and reassure. Council if necessary
Relieved by local heat; change in body position will relieve or reproduce pain	Normal	Examine Reassure. Mild analgesics. Local heat. Rest

Table 4.1 (cont.)

Diagnosis and Character of pain	Location and radiation	Precipitate by or cause
Indigestion Severe burning, sharp dull, aching	Substernally, inframammary to back or abdomen	Lying down, heavy meal exertion/emotion
Liver pain/ cholecystitis		If distended by heart failure, hypoxic or infected
Pulmonary embolism Sudden onset, sharp stabbing, later pleuritic	Substernal, side or back	DVT due to old age, debility, prolonged inactivity, e.g. rest, air travel, leg trauma: right heart disease or pregnancy
Thoracic aortic aneurysm/dissecting Sudden onset, excruciating, tearing sharp pain	Chest, back, abdomen	Sudden exertion. In hypertensive, often elderly people

VENOUS CONGESTION

When the heart chambers become engorged with blood, the pressures within the venous system will rise. Left heart failure will raise the pressure in the left atrium and pulmonary veins to produce dyspnoea. Right heart failure will raise the systemic venous pressures, including the portal system.

Duration or relieved by	Other signs and symptoms	Treatment
May last hours, relieved by antacids, rest or even GTN if due to oesophageal spasm	BP pulse, ECG, and CXR — all normal	Investigations, antacids Change in diet
Variable, last hours Not rest or GTN	If massive, patient collapsed, cyanosed and dyspnotic. If smaller, progressive dyspnoea, followed by pyrexia, cough, haemoptosis and worsening heart failure. ECG tachycardia, ST changes, Q waves in leads II, III and AVF. S waves in leads I and V	Anticoagulants Embolectomy dyspnoeic
Lasts hours, narcotics only	Possibly shocked, anxious. Other symptoms of vessel involvement, carotids, renals or aortic valve. Femoral pulses delayed or absent. CXR may show wide mediasternum	Strict rest, BP control, investigation, aortogram, operation

The liver

The liver will be distended and tender. Pain may be experienced on exercise in some patients. The venous congestion in the liver will impair its function. Jaundice may be present and other liver function tests of serum transminases will be raised, while the erythrocyte sedimentation rate will be reduced. Spider naevi and gynaecomastia may also be present.

Digestion
The gut will also suffer from the raised venous pressure in the portal system causing nausea and anorexia. In some cases of longstanding cardiac failure (e.g. cardiomyopathy) steatorrhoea and protein loss may occur. High venous pressures will cause painful and unsightly varicose veins, or varicose ulcers that will be difficult to heal.

Oedema
The interstitial fluid volume will increase due to the venous pressure exceeding the osmotic pressure in the venules. If concurrent reduction in plasma proteins is present due to poor intake or excessive loss from renal or other disease, the interstitial fluid volume will expand more rapidly (*see* p. 35). Fluid will collect in the tissues of dependent parts of the body. The ankles will swell, initially towards the end of the day, but if the patient is confined to bed the sacrum will show signs of pitting oedema; fluid will not collect in tissues that are drained by gravity, e.g. the face.

Pitting oedema can easily be tested by pressing the fingers gently but firmly into swollen parts of the body. If the skin remains indented then interstitial fluid is excessive. If the cardiac failure or fluid retention is not treated, fluid may further collect in the body cavities to give pleural effusions, abdominal ascites, or a pericardial effusion in severe cases.

Pleural effusions will cause dyspnoea and increase the work of breathing. Pleural aspiration will give instant relief, but the fluid will re-collect if the heart failure is not treated.

Abdominal ascites will be uncomfortable, restrict the patient's movement, and increase anorexia and nausea. Movement of the diaphragm will be restricted, especially if the patient is lying in bed, and thus the work of breathing will increase. Abdominal paracentesis may be necessary to remove the fluid.

A pericardial effusion will restrict the heart's filling capacity, so increasing the venous congestion and lowering the cardiac output. Echocardiography will confirm the presence of the effusion and aspiration will bring dramatic improvement.

DYSPNOEA

This is the principal symptom of left heart failure. Should right heart failure then follow, the degree of dyspnoea will lessen. Symptoms of dyspnoea occur when left atrial pressure rises, e.g. from mitral stenosis or a failing left ventricle. The rise in left atrial pressure will hinder the pulmonary venous flow until the pulmonary venous pressure is higher than the osmotic pressure between capillaries and interstitial lung spaces. Fluid will remain in the lung tissues and some may seep into the alveoli so that the exchange of carbon dioxide and oxygen in the lungs will be reduced. The respiratory centre will thus be stimulated to cause faster and deeper respirations.

These fluid-filled lungs will be less elastic and stiffer to expand, so that more muscular effort is needed to breathe. The sternomastoid muscles will be visible on either side of the neck, the nostrils may flare in an effort to increase air flow, or the patient may mouth breathe. Tracheal tug may be visible in extreme cases. Bronchial veins drain into the pulmonary veins, so that, if these are engorged, the bronchiole lining will swell with oedema causing a dry irritant cough with wheeze.

Any excess fluid in the interstitial spaces or alveoli will be subject to gravity and so normally lie in the lung bases. Crepitations and rales of fluid will be heard by stethoscope and persist after coughing. This fluid, the swollen bronchial mucosa, and the reduced mobility of the patient are the cause of repeated chest infections and winter bronchitis in these patients.

Normally unfit or obese people may be breathless on exertion, but the cardiac patient will report an increase in breathlessness when normal daily activities such as working, walking, or shopping become restricted. In a hospital setting, the nurse can also notice how limited the patient is by dyspnoea. Can he walk briskly around the ward but only slowly upstairs? In extreme cases the patient may be unable to move about the bed or even talk because of breathlessness.

Orthopnea is the need to use several pillows in bed because, if the patient lies flat, he will experience breathlessness. Venous return and cardiac output are increased in the recumbent position, so more fluid is pumped from the right heart into the lungs. Sitting the breathless patient up reduces venous return and right heart output, and re-distributes the fluid to more dependent parts and to the abdominal viscera.

Nocturnal dyspnoea describes the symptom of breathlessness occurring at night as the patient slips down the bed. Such patients may prefer to sleep in a comfortable armchair so that the excess fluid of heart failure stays in the dependent parts of the body, feet, sacrum and lung bases.

Paroxysmal nocturnal dyspnoea (PND)

This describes an acute and frightening occurrence — the patient will suddenly wake up feeling unable to breathe. He will sit up in bed, on the edge of the bed, or stand by an open window in an effort to breathe. PND is caused by the fluid accumulating in the lungs due to left ventricular failure, giving an overwhelming feeling of suffocation. Cardiac asthma is an alternative term used to describe this night time pulmonary oedema because the patient may wheeze and have a dry irritant cough due to the swelling of the bronchial mucosa. Progressive pulmonary oedema will result in frothy oedema fluid being expectorated. This is initially white but, if the pulmonary oedema is severe, the sputum will become pink and frothy due to red cells leaking from the swollen capillaries into the alveoli.

PND is a symptom of severe left ventricular dysfunction. Investigation and treatment (*see* p. 124–6) are necessary otherwise acute and possibly fatal pulmonary oedema may occur.

PALPITATIONS

This is defined as an undue awareness of the heart beat, but does not always indicate heart disease. Anxious persons may be more aware of the heart beat, but the patient with cardiac disease may complain of palpitations where the heart beats very fast, associated with pain, breathlessness, or dizziness.

SYNCOPE

If the cardiac output falls below a level sufficient to maintain cerebral bloodflow, loss of consciousness will occur. Extreme bradycardias or very fast tachycardias (about 300 per minute) may cause unconsciousness in the healthy individual, while lesser disturbances of rhythm with rates of 120 – 180 will cause hypotension and dizziness in those with diseased hearts. Repeated attacks, especially in the elderly, may produce lasting cerebral damage.

The nurse may witness such a syncopal attack or dizzy spell and her observations can greatly aid diagnosis and treatment. A sudden drop in cardiac output sufficient to disturb cerebral bloodflow results in the patient's pulses and blood pressure being difficult or impossible to detect. The skin goes very pale with loss of circulation but, on return of cardiac output, the patient will regain consciousness and the skin will flush pink. Such a description commonly applies to patients with severe aortic stenosis, atrial tumours, or Stokes – Adams attacks from disturbances of cardiac rhythm. The patient may convulse, due to cerebral hypoxia from low bloodflow, but the nurse should definitely distinguish between syncope of cardiac cause and epileptiform fits by the absence or presence of a pulse during the seizure. Transient ischaemia attacks from cerebral artery occlusions or hypoglycaemia can also be differentiated in this way.

Dizziness or unconsciousness may occur with children in tantrums or with adults in excitement or anxiety states who overbreathe; in both however a pulse will be present. Hyperventilation reduces the body carbon dioxide levels which are necessary to maintain cerebral bloodflow.

Obstruction to bloodflow

A massive pulmonary embolism may stop blood from the right heart reaching the left heart; unconsciousness and death may follow. Similarly an atrial tumour — a myxoma — grows on a pedicle so that, with certain positions of the patient, the tumour may block the atrioventricular valve, causing syncope and loss of pulse. The tumour will usually move away from the valve as the person faints, but this may not always occur, so the long term prognosis is poor unless the tumour is detected by echocardiography and surgically excised.

Partial obstruction to bloodflow within the heart and lungs may cause syncope on exertion, i.e. when the skeletal muscles demand a greater bloodflow than can pass the occlusion to supply the muscles and the brain. Possible causes of this condition include Fallot's tetralogy, severe pulmonary hypertension, severe aortic stenosis, and hypertrophic obstructive cardiomyopathy (HOCM). Episodes of syncope should be urgently investigated, meanwhile sudden exertion should be avoided.

Postural hypotension

When a person stands up from the lying position, blood flows to the areas of low pressure in the leg arterioles. This occurs at the expense of cerebral bloodflow unless the peripheral arterioles compensate by constricting. Patients who have been on prolonged bed rest lose this peripheral vascular control, and care is needed when first getting these patients up. Leg exercises, flexing the leg muscles, or swinging the legs while sitting on the edge of the bed, will prevent sudden hypotension and dizziness. Venous return and hence cardiac output can thereby be increased.

Those receiving drugs to block the alpha adrenergic responses to treat hypertension may also experience a fall in blood pressure on standing (orthostatic hypotension). Elderly patients who require treatment for hypertension may also have disease of cerebral blood vessels and therefore these drugs are not suitable for them. Chlorpromazine has a similar vasodilating effect.

Increased vagal tone

Syncope may ocur in an otherwise healthy but susceptible person due to
increased vagal stimulation such as unpleasant sights or distressing news.
Initial bradycardia is followed by tachycardia and the skin becomes pale
and sweaty due to a sudden reduction in peripheral vascular resistance.
Recovery occurs soon after the person falls or lies down, but the pallor and
fatigue may last for several hours.

Stimulation of the carotid sinus, straining at stool, or emptying a full
bladder (especially in elderly people) may increase vagal tone and cause
faintness. This may be useful to treat a tachycardia by, for example,
rubbing the carotid sinus, pressing the eyeballs, or performing the
Valsalva manoeuvre. These may be so effective in reducing vagal tone that
extreme bradycardia or asystole can occur. However, in appropriate cases
of tachyarrhythmias, the Valsalva manoeuvre is used under medical
supervision: ask the patient to try to breathe out against a closed glottis.
This raises the intrathoracic pressure in the same way as straining at stool
and vagal tone will increase as a result, slowing the heart rate (sometimes
drastically). It should thus only be done under medical supervision.

SYSTEMIC EMBOLI

Thrombus can form in the left heart when stasis of blood occurs in dilated
or poorly contracting chambers, due to hypertrophy, infarction, aneursym
formation, or atrial fibrillation. The roughened endothelial surface of
infarction necrosis or infection allows platelets to aggregate. Valves
damaged by rheumatic fever and bacterial endocarditis develop infected
fibrin formations called vegetations which can break loose and embolize,
to cause organ necrosis and abscesses. Emboli from the left heart can
travel to any artery to cause death of tissue; the site and size of any artery
obstructed will give rise to a variety of symptoms.

Micro-emboli may cause petechial haemorrhages on the skin, possibly
unnoticed by the patient, but seen by the nurse when washing him.
Splinter haemorrhages in the nail bed are often the first sign of the micro-
emboli of endocarditis.

TREATMENT OF HEART FAILURE

All patients with signs or symptoms of heart failure should be investigated
to establish the underlying cause and its severity. Treating the disease
process directly is not always possible (e.g. cardiomyopathy) nor always
advisable (e.g. operating on every patient with mild valve disease).

Medical therapy to aid the failing heart is aimed at improving contractility either directly or, more importantly, indirectly in several ways which include: **1** reversing the known causes or aggravating factors where possible, **2** reducing the workload on the myocardium (using rest, digitalis, diuretics and vasodilators), and **3** stimulating the myocardium with drugs. These will now be discussed in turn.

Reversing the cause of poor myocardial contraction

To achieve this, acidosis should be treated with sodium bicarbonate and electrolytes of potassium and calcium should be brought to within normal limits. Hypoxia may be due to lung disease or pulmonary oedema where the arterial oxygen levels will be low. Giving the patient oxygen to breathe could greatly improve his cardiac condition. However, patients with myocardial ischaemia due to coronary artery disease or ischaemic cardiomyopathy will have normal arterial blood oxygen, and an oxygen mask may be more of a nuisance than a help.

Reducing the workload on the myocardium — preload

REST

This can effectively improve cardiac function because, with the reduction in muscular activity, venous return will be reduced. The smaller volume of blood returning to the heart will reduce the filling pressure (preload) on the dilated, failing ventricles. These less full ventricles will now be able to empty themselves more thoroughly at each systole, so reducing the diastolic pressure within the ventricles. This reduction in intraventricular pressures will allow the overstretched muscle fibres to again overlap each other in the normal manner. Cavity size will return to normal, the heart will work more effectively, and cardiac output will rise.

The improvement can be shown by the reduced size of the heart shadow on chest X-ray and by the slowing of the rapid heart rate that was previously necessary to maintain cardiac output in the presence of poor contractility.

Renal bloodflow will also improve with rest. In the presence of low cardiac output, blood will be diverted to exercising muscles at the expense of the peripheries, gut, and kidneys. With rest, blood will not be required in great quantities by the muscles so bloodflow to the kidneys will improve. Urine output will increase so relieving preload and oedema. This improvement in renal function can be measured by a fall in the patient's weight and reduction in oedema.

DIGITALIS

Digitalis is a very ancient drug which greatly aids the failing heart — up to a limit — but which does not improve contractility in normal hearts. Although we do not yet fully understand why and how digitalis improves heart muscle contraction, we do know that it increases the ability of the actin and myocin filaments to stretch and shorten, so improving cardiac contraction directly. This also increases the effects of rest which are described above.

Digitalis will produce a dramatic improvement in the patients with atrial fibrillation by lengthening the refractory times of atrial and AV node tissue; hence fewer impulses will reach the ventricles and ventricular rate will slow. A slower, more regular heart rate will reduce heart work and improve cardiac output. Many patients will revert to sinus rhythm.

Dosage
Oral digoxin (the commonly used form of digitalis) will slow a tachycardia in 4 – 6 hours. Intravenous digoxin, 0.5 mg given over 10 minutes can be used to slow the heart rate in urgent situations. The potassium level should be checked prior to its administration. Toxic effects of digitalis, especially in the presence of hypokalaemia, can be very dangerous. Dosage is carefully calculated, taking into account the patient's age and renal function. The initial dosage is 0.5 mg × 2 or 3 doses 6 hourly and 0.25 mg b.d. thereafter. Elderly patients, or those with renal impairment, will be given smaller doses e.g. 0.25 mg 12 hourly × 2 doses, then 0.125 mg on alternate days. Antacids disturb the absorption of digoxin.

Toxicity
This can be very dangerous. Cardiac rhythm may become erractic, changing in the same patient from ventricular bigeminy, junctional rhythm, and atrioventricular blocks, to rapid atrial flutter or fibrillation all in one hour. Fortunately other signs and symptoms occur before the cardiac ones, so the drug can be stopped and serum levels checked. Some symptoms can be difficult to differentiate from the symptoms of the heart failure: lethargy, anorexia, nausea, or vomiting; however, digoxin toxicity causes visual disturbances and diarrhoea.

DIURETICS

In the reduction of the workload of the myocardium, diuretics are used in conjunction with several other therapeutic approaches including rest, fluid restriction and salt restriction. The more common drugs are:

Frusemide	Tabs. 40 – 160 mg or i.v. 20 – 250 mg
Bumetanide	1 – 4 mg per day: i.m. 1 – 2 mg or i.v. 2 – 5 mg over 30 – 60 minutes
Ethacrynic acid	25 – 125 mg: i.v. 50 mg slowly

These potent diuretics reduce the amount of sodium re-absorbed at the loop of Henle, hence more salt and water are lost in the urine. A rapid diuresis occurs, even in patients with severe oedema, beginning after one hour and lasting for about six hours. Tablets are prescribed in the morning to promote an early diuresis but, if tablets are given in the evening, they should be timed for 3 – 4 hours before sleep is planned, to allow the patient to pass all the urine formed before he retires to bed. Evening diuretics may be prescribed for patients who experience nocturnal dyspnoea.

Intravenous injection of these diuretics gives an almost instant effect and can be used in the acutely ill patient. A massive diuresis may occur which may reduce venous return so severely that cardiac output could fall. The plasma urea levels may rise in aggressive diuretic therapy, and gout and diabetes can be precipitated. Very large doses may be given to patients in renal failure, and deafness may occur.

Thiaziades

| Cyclopenthiazide *(Navidrex)* | 0.25 – 1 mg daily |
| Bendrofluazide | 2.5 – 10 mg daily |

These drugs inhibit the re-absorbtion of sodium in the ascending loop of Henle and the distal convoluted tubule. Skin rashes and bone marrow depression occur rarely.

Thiazides are effective when used once daily for patients in mild or moderate heart failure or hypertension. Onset of action occurs after 1 – 2 hours and lasts for 12 – 24 hours.

Potassium depletion with diuretics

When salt and water excretion are increased, potassium is also lost from the body with resulting muscle weakness and myocardial irritability. In addition, a particular danger of potassium depletion is that digoxin toxicity can be accelerated. To combat this, oral supplements of potassium are given usually as sugar-coated slow-release tablets since the effervescent preparations can irritate the intestinal mucosa to produce nausea, vomiting and ulceration. The usual dose of Slow K tablets is 2 t.d.s., but preparations are made with the diuretic and potassium within one tablet, e.g. Navidrex K.

As an alternative to supplements, the patient can be encouraged to eat potassium-rich foods, such as bananas, fresh orange juice, or chocolate. However, patients on intravenous fluids only, especially those receiving diuretic therapy, will need intravenous potassium which is a concentrated preparation and, if given in a bolus, would cause ventricular fibrillation. It should be diluted and given slowly via a central line, i.e. no faster than 10 mmol over 15 – 20 minutes. If a strong solution of potassium in an infusion extravasates into the tissues, necrosis can occur.

Aldosterone antagonists
Aldactone A is given 25 – 50 mg t.d.s. either alone or with a thiazide. Amiloride 5 – 10 mg reduces the potassium and hydrogen ion exchange in the distal tubules when given with each dose of diuretic. Take care not to increase potassium levels with these two drugs as they are very effective in preventing potassium loss.

Reducing the workload on the myocardium — afterload

Since the heart must work harder to eject blood at systole in the presence of increased resistance, removal of the obstruction or resistance will relieve the failing heart so enabling it to empty itself completely and effectively into the arteries. Treatment is therefore concentrated on this aspect according to the specific cause of heart failure: valve stenosis is treated with valvotomy or replacement, hypertension is treated in acute or longstanding cases, acute vasoconstriction is treated by vasodilation, and coarctation of the aorta is treated by operation to remove the stricture.

VASODILATION

Vasodilation relieves the afterload on the heart and leads to an increase in the intravascular compartment which makes ejection of blood at systole easier. Cardiac output will rise and bloodflow to tissues will increase. Blood pressure remains the same or falls (*see* Fig. 2.12).

This treatment can therefore be used to alleviate hypertension and, if the fluid retention which is so common with hypertensive disease is removed with diuretics at the same time, the venous return to the heart will fall. Blood pressure and cardiac output will also fall with possibly undesirable consequences. Thus, in the treatment of hypertension, diuresis and vasodilation must be balanced to produce a fall in systolic and diastolic pressures without causing side-effects of dizziness or syncope.

The shocked patient may also benefit from vasodilation. The reduction in afterload will increase bloodflow to the tissues and kidneys so reversing tissue hypoxia, acidosis, and impending renal failure. However, despite the fact that the reduction in afterload enables the failing heart to produce a bigger cardiac output with less effort, improvement will *not* be an initial rise in blood pressure, but increased tissue perfusion, i.e. warmer, dryer skin, increased urine output, and improved conscious level. A reduction in heart rate will follow as the stroke volume increases.

SYMPATHETIC TONE

Vasoconstriction will occur if sympathetic tone is increased. To prevent this, or to effect a vasodilation, drugs can be given which block the receptors at the sympathetic nerve endings. The transmitter at these nerve endings is noradrenaline, hence the action of catecholamines released by the adrenal medulla or of intravenous adrenaline will be blocked by these drugs, which fall into two main categories: alpha and beta adrenergic receptor blockers.

Alpha receptor blockers remove sympathetic tone to arteries and veins in muscles and to peripheral vessels. Vasodilation, with a fall in CVP and reduction in blood pressure, will result. Unfortunately, orthostatic hypotension is a problem with these drugs so they are not used routinely for treating hypertension. However, they are very effective in a hypertensive crisis and can be used to control the blood pressure problems of phaeochromocytoma. A reflex tachycardia usually occurs.

Two common preparations are phentolamine (Rogitine) 5 – 10 mg bolus i.v. and phenoxybenzamine (Dibenyline) i.v. 50 mg, orally 20 – 100 mg.

Beta receptor blockers block beta stimulation to the heart and other areas. Heart rate, conduction, irritability, and contractility will be reduced (with possible consequent heart failure); cardiac output and blood pressure will fall; and demand for myocardial oxygen will fall. These drugs are therefore particularly effective for treating angina. Blood pressure is lowered by a number of mechanisms including a reduction in plasma renin and a central effect on the vasomotor centre with some drugs. A number of patients experience vivid dreams and hallucinations.

Three common preparations are propranalol 40 – 160 mg t.d.s., 1 mg i.v. over one minute, oxprenolol 20 – 100 mg t.d.s., 1 – 2 mg i.v. slowly, and pindolol 7.5 – 45 mg in one day.

Because all beta receptors will be blocked, patients with asthma, bronchitis, or peripheral vascular disease should be given a cardioselective beta blocking agent such as metoprolol (100 – 400 mg orally in one day, or 5 mg i.v. given over 5 – 10 minutes), practolol (5 mg i.v. slowly. Not used orally now as it caused peritoneal fibrosis and conjunctival scarring in long term use), or labetalol (300 mg – 2.4 g daily orally, or 50 mg i.v. over one minute or up to 200 mg by infusion at 2 mg/minute). The latter is an alpha and beta blocking agent and effectively reduces blood pressure.

CENTRALLY ACTING DRUGS

Methyldopa (Aldomet)
250 mg – 1 g orally t.d.s.

Diuretics are frequently used with this drug to control moderate to severe hypertension or a hypertensive crisis. Side-effects include a dry mouth, sedation or depression, diarrhoea, fluid retention, and failure of ejaculation.

Clonidine (Catapres)
50 – 400 µg t.d.s. or 150 – 300 µg by slow i.v. injection

This is given to treat moderate to severe hypertension. Side-effects include dry mouth, sedation, depression, fluid retention, bradycardia and Raynaud's phenomenon. Sudden withdrawal of this drug will result in a hypertensive crisis, so patients must be urged to take their tablets regularly.

POTENT VASODILATORS

Glyceryl trinitrate (GTN)
0.5 mg sublingually as required

These tablets cause widespread vasodilation of arteries and especially the veins for 2 – 3 minutes. This offloads the heart and reduces preload, therefore less heart work is required. Angina is relieved because the heart has less work to do, its own oxygen requirements will be reduced, hence the amount of blood flowing through the diseased coronary arteries will be adequate for the heart muscle needs (*see* Angina, p.182).

Nitroglycerine paste
1 – 2 inches t.d.s.

The paste is placed on the skin under a piece of paper, commonly on the chest wall or abdomen, and is absorbed over several hours to produce vasodilation. It is used to treat angina and heart failure.

Isosorbide
Tabs. 10 mg t.d.s.
Sublingual 5 mg 2 hourly and as required

Intravenous infusion 10 – 50 mg in 500 ml

This has a similar action as GTN only the effect is more potent and lasts longer. The sublingual preparation is effective almost immediately and, apart from angina relief, it is used to reduce the work of the failing heart. The tablets can be taken regularly to prevent angina, but the effect is not as good as the sublingual preparation.

Intravenous isosorbide is given to patients in acute heart failure and cardiogenic shock via a continuous infusion. Vasodilation with a reduction in heart work will result. This drug also dilates veins and the pulmonary arteries, so that preload to the right and left heart will be reduced; pulmonary vascular resistance will fall producing a reduction in afterload for the right ventricle for patients with right heart failure and pulmonary hypertension.

Nitroprusside (Nipride)
50 – 100 mg in 500 ml infusion

This potent vasodilator rapidly reduces arterial and venous pressures. It is used to treat hypertensive patients at risk and also those in cardiogenic shock, where reduction in afterload is urgently required. In these shocked patients nitroprusside is commonly used in conjunction with adrenaline to override the dangerous tissue and renal constriction caused by adrenaline.

This drug should be given via an infusion pump and the solution freshly prepared every six hours as it can degenerate into a blue infusion of cyanide, if exposed to sunlight. This degeneration is reduced if the solution is protected from sunlight.

Hydralazine (Apresoline)
10 – 20 mg bolus i.v. or 25 – 100 mg b.d. orally
This is used in heart failure and in moderate or severe hypertension, commonly in conjunction with beta blocking agents or a thiazide diuretic. If given intravenously a rapid drop in blood pressure and CVP will result. Side-effects include postural hypotension, tachycardia, nausea, and vomiting.

Diazoxide (Eudemine)
300 mg by rapid i.v. injection

This can be used to vasodilate and lower the blood pressure in a hypertensive crisis. It should not be used for patients with renal disease, coronary artery disease, or pregnancy because its side-effects include hyperglycaemia, fluid retention, and tachycardia.

Nifedipine (Adalat)
10 – 20 mg t.d.s. or for immediate action the capsule can be bitten and the fluid kept in the mouth.

This has a specific action on the coronary arteries and peripheral vessels. It is therefore used in treatment of angina and coronary spasm.

Cardiac stimulants

Dobutamine
Infusion 250 mg – 1 g in 500 ml
5 – 20 μg/kg/minute

This drug has a more specific action on contractility than either isoprenaline or adrenaline, and it also dilates renal arteries. This double effect makes it a most useful drug in low cardiac output and hypotensive states as these impair renal perfusion. However in high doses dopamine has an almost pure noradrenaline effect on the heart and arteries so causing tachycardia and vasoconstriction with a rise in blood pressure but a fall in renal perfusion. Dopamine is usually given via an infusion pump, and patients can be slowly weaned from this support over hours or days.

Dobutamine
Infusion 250 mg – 1 g in 500 ml
2.5 – 10 μg/kg/minute

This drug has a similar action on the heart as dopamine, but causes less tachycardia. It improves contractility and hence stroke volume. Tachycardia and hypertension are signs of overdosage.

It is usually given via an infusion pump and patients are slowly weaned from this over a period of hours.

Noradrenaline
8 – 10 μg/minute i.v. infusion or 100 – 150 μg bolus

Adrenaline
i.v. bolus 1 : 10 000 1 – 10 ml
i.v. infusion 10 – 40 mg in 500 ml

Noradrenaline is responsible for the transmission at the end of sympathetic nerves. Noradrenaline and adrenaline can be released by the adrenal medulla to mimic sympathetic stimulation; they can also be given intravenously. Sympathetic stimulation on the heart will cause increases in the following: sinus rate (heart rate), AV conduction, myocardial contractility (stroke volume), myocardial irritability. It will also cause vasoconstriction (i.e. blood pressure and afterload increased) and bronchodilation.

Adrenaline is used more than noradrenaline and is usually reserved for very serious bradycardias or hypotensive episodes, and to restore cardiac action following cardiac arrest. It has a potent action to increase heart rate and contraction, but the increase in peripheral resistance from the concurrent vasoconstriction is desirable only until extreme hypotension is reversed. Nitroprusside may be given simultaneously to override the vasoconstriction or low dose dopamine given to maintain renal bloodflow.

Isoprenaline (beta receptor stimulator)
Bolus 200 μg
Infusion 5 mg in 500 ml at 0.5 – 10 μg per minute

Isoprenaline does not naturally occur in the body but it has similar properties to adrenaline. It acts only on beta receptors, hence it causes an increase in heart rate, conduction, contractility or irritability with less vasoconstriction than adrenaline.

It is given by bolus or infusion to treat serious bradycardias, heart blocks, and low cardiac output states.

Calcium chloride
This electrolyte is essential for muscle contraction, and the movement of ions across the cell membrane in re-polarization.

In the event of a cardiac arrest, it can be given as a bolus with adrenaline and may restore heart action. In hypotensive or low output states, it may improve stroke volume when given over 5 – 10 minutes. If given too fast, asystole may occur.

NURSING INTERVENTION FOR CHRONIC OR MILD HEART FAILURE

The well-informed nurse can contribute much to aid the diagnosis and treatment of this condition, particularly since, although diuretics, vasodilators, and cardiac stimulant drugs may be used, diet and rest are at least as important.

Rest

Rest, or a reduction in activities, is essential until the heart failure is controlled, if basic tissue oxygen requirements are to be met (*see* p. 105). Rest alone can tide the body over a critical all in cardiac output, allowing blood to flow to essential organs instead of exercising muscles. In addition, a reduction in a fast heart rate will usually reduce heart work and myocardial oxygen needs, therefore tachycardia-producing events (such as exertion, pain, or anxiety (*see below*)) should be avoided.

The hospital regime should be organized with this need in mind. Visitors should be seen by the nursing staff and advised of the patient's need to rest. Prolonged visiting by even close family may excessively tire or worry the patient; the nurse must use her discretion when to encourage or discourage visiting.

The plan of rest will vary from patient to patient and should be discussed with the individual to achieve understanding and compliance with this treatment. Patients who have mild heart failure may only be admitted for a few days for investigations and obviously do not require bed rest; however, when they go home and back to work, it should be made clear that a general reduction in activities will be beneficial. More time should be spent quietly resting, if possible after lunch, in the evening and at weekends. Though the patient may have to rearrange his pattern of life a little, it does not mean that he should totally shun social entertainments or work commitments. For the severely ill patient, bed rest may be necessary, but he should be allowed up to use a commode or bottle and to sit in a chair for short periods.

ANXIETY

Florence Nightingale said, 'Apprehension, waiting, expectation, fear of surprise do a patient more harm than any exertion.' The nurse can contribute greatly to a cardiac patient's recovery by relieving any anxiety or pain, for unexplained pain may be a major factor contributing to an anxiety tachycardia.

Anxiety relief can begin before the patient is first admitted. Many hospitals send information leaflets to booked admissions which explain the uniforms and role of various hospital staff, visiting times, hospital services of social worker, library, hair dressing and shopping facilities. Special thought must be given to the emergency admission or transfer patient who will not have had this preparation.

On admission, the patient and relatives should be welcomed and introduced to relevant ward personnel, the ward layout and times of meals, doctors' visits, visiting hours, and to neighbouring patients in a friendly, respectful, and professional manner — which should all help the patient to feel at ease. To prevent the patient and family worrying unnecessarily, they should be encouraged to ask questions about any aspect of the hospital stay. Despite this, some patients may develop anxiety tachycardias because of concerns at home, at work, or even about neighbouring patients. The observant nurse should be able to elucidate problems of this kind when she talks and listens to the patient while carrying out procedures and when taking the nursing history. Explanation of the cause of any pains or discomfort (e.g. liver congestion or angina) may reassure the patient that, although the pains are related to the heart disease, they should be relieved with treatment. Calm and unhurried explanation prior to any procedure or investigation should prevent the patient developing anxiety tachycardias or dangerous arrhythmias.

SLEEP

Sleep will obviously reduce body oxygen requirements, and many cardiologists prescribe day and night time sedation. Sleep will also help the patient suffering from lethargy and despondency who may not have slept well for weeks.

The discomfort from an enlarged liver, ascites or a troublesome dry cough may prevent the patient receiving adequate sleep. Periods during the day should be designated as rest periods. Reduction in noise and light as well as grouping of disturbances, nursing activities, meals, and doctors' visits should be planned to allow periods of uninterrupted rest.

LETHARGY

Tiredness is a feature of many illnesses and can be due to lack of sleep caused by other symptoms or the disease itself. Lethargy is common in low cardiac output states and is particularly marked in mitral incompetence. Electrolyte imbalance from diuretic therapy may cause muscle weakness and cramp. The patient will tire easily, will need to sit down frequently, and may find even non-exertional aspects of daily living or housework exhausting.

Possible complications of bed rest

The reduced blood flow to the skin and extremities will cause them to be cool and cyanosed. The patients will complain that their hands, and particularly their feet, feel cold even in bed. Wearing woollen socks will obviously help.

The risk of *pressure necrosis* is great with lower skin perfusion, and interstitial oedema. Meticulous attention is therefore needed in the care of the skin. Patients should be encouraged to change their position in bed at least two hourly, though the ill patients will require two nurses to move them if they are to avoid undue exertion. Patients at risk should be nursed with sheep skins under their heels and buttocks to prevent direct constant pressure to one area. To prevent discomfort on oedematous legs, ascites, or a distended liver, the bedding should be warm but light; a quilt is ideal and available in some hospitals, otherwise the use of bed cradles is necessary to support heavy blankets. Free movement of the legs must be possible, and two hourly active leg exercises should be encouraged or passive exercises for the seriously ill to prevent venous stasis.

Patients with reduced circulation with high venous pressures are at risk of developing *venous stasis*. Varicose veins may become more prominent and uncomfortable, varicose ulcers may develop and will be difficult to heal. Deep vein thrombosis is a real risk, especially if the patient is confined to bed or spends much of the day in a chair. Multiple small emboli may break away to lodge in the lungs, producing pleuritic pain, haemoptysis or pleural effusions. These lung emboli will contribute to pulmonary hypertension, right heart failure, and reduced lung function. Prophylactic anticoagulants may be given, especially to the obese. Subcutaneous heparin 5000 units t.d.s. may be prescribed, however those patients in atrial fibrillation or with large hearts and ventricular aneurysms may already be prescribed oral anticoagulation with warfarin. Other patients with angina or myocardial infarction are not routinely anticoagulated, though this subject remains controversial after many years of research.

A chest infection or hypostatic pneumonia is a risk in immobile patients, especially those with heart failure as there will be an increase in interstitial lung fluid. Deep breathing and coughing exercises should be encouraged two hourly to prevent atelectasis. Active physiotherapy or steam inhalations are not usually necessary unless the chest infection becomes a serious component of the illness. A Bird or Bennet respirator may be cautiously used, but great care is needed with bronchodilators because these cause tachycardias. Tipping with percussion and strenuous vibration will be very tiring physically and should only be used when absolutely necessary, and then under medical supervision.

DYSPNOEA

If the patient experiences sudden breathlessness and is anxious but not shocked, the nurse should reassure him, keep him within view, and give him a nurse-call bell. Sitting the patient up in bed, well supported on pillows, will often bring relief. The patient may prefer to sit on the edge of the bed and lean over a bed table. Many patients, especially the obese or those with coexisting respiratory disease, may be more comfortable sitting and even sleeping in an armchair than in bed. The administration of oxygen sometimes helps, possibly as a psychological support rather than for physiological need for mild cardiac dyspnoea.

The nurse should observe the patient and record observations of temperature, respirations, blood pressure and heart rate, noting especially if the heart rhythm has changed or become irregular. The patient's fluid balance status should be noted, intake and weight may be increased and urine output down if the patient is retaining fluid. The frequency of these attacks, their precipitating and relieving factors and any other symptoms should be documented in the nursing records and the doctor informed.

Treatment
Diuretics and digoxin may be started or increased and beta blocking agents reduced. Any pleural effusions may be aspirated and antibiotics stated if a chest infection is suspected. Severe dyspnoea may require intravenous diamorphine, frusemide, aminophylline and possibly vasodilators or cardiac stimulants. If the patient has an arrhythmia (e.g. supraventricular tachycardia) this may be the cause of the attack of left ventricular failure. Anti-arrhythmics will be given and the patient possibly transferred to a monitoring unit.

INTESTINAL DISTURBANCE AND DIET

A particular source of discomfort and misery to patients with mild cardiac failure is produced by the low perfusion, venous congestion, and reduced mobility of the gut. The diet should be light, appetising and easily digestible. If low animal fat or reducing diets are needed, these can be introduced after the first few days. Many patients are anorexic initially and may request fluids only for 24 – 48 hours. Any dietary requests should be catered for as far as possible, including those families who may wish to bring in special foods for those with cultural or religious customs and rules affecting their diet.

Cardiac cachexia
It is important that the gut is also rested in long term failure. The loss of appetite and reduction in activities may produce severe muscle and fat wastage. The patient will have a gaunt face and thin arms. If severe fluid

retention with dependent oedema and abdominal acites are present, the extent of the wasting may not be obvious until after effective diuretic therapy.

Salt restriction
Salt restriction in the diet will reduce total body water and sodium, but food cooked without salt is tasteless and unappetizing, especially for the already anorexic patient. With the use of potent salt-losing diuretics it is not necessary to severely restrict salt in cooking, but salty foods such as kippers should be avoided and salt should not be added after food has been cooked.

Fluid restriction
Salt and fluid restriction should be discussed with the patient. Patients receiving diuretics will become very thirsty. Between 1000 and 1500 ml a day are common restrictions for an adult, and the patient can be helped to adhere to this amount by dividing the allowance between meal and tea break times, allowing water for tablets and night time. Half cups of tea, if drunk slowly, may be almost as satisfying as whole cups. Give only a small water glass to the patient and offer frequent mouth washes. These plans should prevent the patient drinking all his allowance by lunch time.

Fluid balance charts are important in the ill patient to assess progress, but daily weighing at the same time each day is less restrictive for the patient and will clearly indicate if the patient is losing or gaining oedema fluid. The patient with chronic cardiac disease who will be maintained on large doses of diuretics should be encouraged to manage his own fluid intake and balance in preparation for when he goes home.

Abdominal ascites will produce a full feeling for the patient, who may mistake the fluid swelling for obesity and be reluctant to eat. The patient may find eating difficult or tiring even when well supported on pillows; therefore the ill patients may be better sat out of bed for meals.

Constipation
Most analgesics have a constipating effect so that aperients are usually necessary to prevent constipation until the patient is ambulant. Straining at stool should be discouraged as it increases intrathoracic pressure (the Valsalva manoeuvre), so increasing vagal tone and possibly causing extreme bradycardia post myocardial infarction. All but the very seriously ill patient may use the bedside commode. Constipation can cause discomfort, anorexia, nausea and even vomiting. Dorbanex nocte (*Riker*) may not be sufficient and, if constipation has been a longstanding problem

with heart failure, suppositories or an enema may be needed.

To increase appetite and absorption, anti-emetics may be prescribed before meals and with each dose of any narcotic analgesia to prevent nausea. Appetisers of stout or sherry may be very effective, if only for their calorie content and sedative effect. A diet of only nourishing fluids may not be possible if the patient is on a fluid intake restriction.

To digest a heavy meal, bloodflow to the gut must increase; the heart will thus have a larger output demanded of it. This is why patients experience angina if they exert themselves even only slightly after a meal and why a rest after meals is advisable.

Patient observation

Dyspnoea, chest pains, palpitations and oedema are often the cause of the patient's admission to a cardiac ward, however syncope and systemic emboli may also be of cardiac origin. The exact cause of the symptoms and signs in a particular patient may not be clear. Diagnosis can be greatly aided by the detailed description from a witness of an episode of one of these symptoms.

SYNCOPE

The cardiac patient may complain of dizziness of faintness, but occasionally loss of consciousness may occur. This syncope may be due to not enough oxygenated blood perfusing the brain, either from a dramatic fall or cessation of cardiac output, or from narrowed carotid arteries. Loss of consciousness can also occur with hypoglycaemia or epileptiform fits.

If the pulse remains of good volume and rate, but the patient is dizzy or unconscious, the cause of the attack is *not* from a low cardiac output.

Nursing intervention

Assess the patient's condition. If he is unconscious and pulseless, commence the cardiac arrest procedure immediately. If he is not in cardiac arrest or he quickly regains pulse and then consciousness, lie the patient down, stay with him, assess his conscious level, and alert the medical staff. Feel for the volume, rate, and rhythm of the pulse, noting if there are any irregularities.

Observe the skin colour. A cessation in cardiac output will cause the patient to go deathly pale, then to flush bright pink when the cardiac output returns. Note also if the patient is breathless, has any chest pain or any signs of muscular twitching or paralysis. Has the patient been incontinent? As soon as possible record a monitor rhythm tracing or a 12 lead ECG.

Assist the patient into a comfortable position, tell him that he had fainted. Ask him to describe how he felt before the attack, and also what exactly he was doing just before he fainted.

The doctor will examine the patient for cardiac signs, and also for any injuries that might have occurred due to the patient falling, e.g. a head or limb injury. The doctor will question any nurse who witnessed the syncopal episode, with particular reference as to whether a pulse was present or not, and he will look at a recent ECG.

Depending on these findings the doctor may institute the following.
1 Transfer the patient to a monitoring unit or arrange for ambulatory monitoring.
2 Arrange for the insertion of a temporary or permanent pacing wire.
3 Insert an intravenous line and administer atropine, adrenaline or isoprenaline (for bradycardias or heart blocks) or anti-arrhythmic drugs (for supraventricular tachycardia or numerous ectopics which indicate the syncope may have been due to a ventricular tachycardia).
4 Alter the dosage of diuretics, beta blocking agents, or other hypotensive agents.
5 If the syncope may have been caused by a cardiac lesion (e.g. aortic stenosis), arrange early investigation and instruct the patient to rest.
6 If the attack was not cardiac in origin (i.e. a good pulse was present throughout the attack) the cause must be found. The doctor will take blood for blood sugar levels, take X-rays of the neck, and carry out a neurological examination (possibly including carotid angiograms)

SYSTEMIC EMBOLI

An awareness of those at risk from emboli will help the nurse to observe for signs of small skin petechial haemorrhages, blood in the urine and signs of cerebral and limb involvement, often noticed during bathing.

Investigations and treatment
A full medical examination and history may reveal signs of the source of the emboli. ECG, echocardiography, chest X-ray and blood cultures may be taken. If atrial fibrillation, heart failure or a ventricular aneursym are present, long term anticoagulants may be prescribed, as well as specific treatments.

An embolism to a limb or the mesentary will require urgent surgery or i.v. heparinization or streptokinase (a thrombolytic agent) may be indicated. If active endocarditis is suspected, vigorous antibiotic therapy will begin after blood cultures have been taken. Urgent cardiac surgery may be indicated to remove a diseased valve or a clot-filled ventricular aneursym.

Table 4.2 Nursing care for heart failure

Problem	Aim	Plan
Low cardiac output, myocardial overload	Improve cardiac function	REST — physical and mental
Poor peripheral perfusion, pressure sore risk, cold peripheries	No pressure sores, warmer peripheries	Light bedding/skin care, sheepskins. Change position 2 hourly
Venous stasis, deep vein thrombosis risk	No DVT or pulmonary emboli	Light bedding/leg exercises, early mobilization. ? anticoagulation
Reduced gut motility, anorexia, malnutrition, constipation	Improve appetite, adequate nutrition, relieve constipation	Discuss diet with patient, antiemetics, appetisers, light nourishing diet, aperients
Pulmonary congestion Hypostatic pneumonia risk	No chest infection	Deep breathing and coughing exercises. Early mobilization
Lethargy Despondency	Restore energy and interest in life	Rest and sleep. Information & involvement with own care. Occupational therapy
Fluid retention Oedema	Loss of oedema fluid	Rest. Salt and water intake restriction. Weigh daily
Electrolyte imbalance, muscle weakness	Normal electrolytes	Balance fluids and diet, care with minerals, especially potassium

Mobilization

When the heart rate, oedema, heart size and other symptoms and signs are all responding to treatment, more physical activity will be encouraged. The patient who has been in severe heart failure will start mobilizing very gently. He can be wheeled to the toilet and bathroom and assisted with bathing initially, gradually building up activities until he can walk round the ward aided by a physiotherapist or nurse and eat his meals at the table. Periods of rest on or in the bed will be necessary and the speed of mobilization will be guided by the patient's feeling of well being, his pulse rate, heart and chest sounds, and any signs or symptoms of recurring heart failure.

The patient will probably have been feeling lethargic due to a low cardiac output, and may begin to feel full of energy and vigour as his condition improves. Guidelines to activities in the ward and on returning home should be given, otherwise heart failure may be exacerbated. Guidelines similar to those for patients following myocardial infarction should be given (*see* p. 198), though it should be stressed that each person will respond to treatment differently. Some patients may have to accept continuing restrictions on their daily activities if heart failure can only be contained, e.g. those with cardiomyopathy or extensive myocardial infarction. Patients who have only mild heart failure that has responded well to therapy can return to a full and normal life. Advice concerning strenuous activities, diet, smoking and rest should be tailored to the individual patient.

Chapter 5
Severe heart failure

Every hospital that has a casualty, coronary care unit or is a specialized cardiac referral hospital, should have facilities for receiving patients with acute cardiac problems. All resources should be readily available. Nursing staff should know how to involve other personnel and how to prepare and use equipment. They will thus be the basis of an effective working team capable of receiving and treating any cardiac emergency.

On arrival, the patient will be in a state of extreme anxiety about his condition; reception by a calm but efficient cardiac team can greatly relieve this feeling. If pulmonary oedema is present the patient will be extremely anxious, restless, dyspnoeic, hypoxic and will expectorate copious frothy sputum. With the minimum of delay and fuss make the patient comfortable, lying in a head-up position in bed (or on the casualty trolley). Attach the patient to the cardiac monitor, administer oxygen by a mask or nasal cannulae, and prepare for the insertion of an intravenous cannula.

Nurses have an important role, not only in caring for the patient's comfort and observing his condition but in skilfully and completely resting the patient to aid the heart to meet tissue oxygen needs.

ASSESSMENT

To assess the patient's condition, take the normal observations and recordings of temperature, heart rate, respiration, and blood pressure. A 12 lead ECG and monitor rhythm tracing should be recorded.

More important than these recordings is the recognition of any physiological mechanisms that are causing or compensating for the low cardiac output state. These include a raised sympathetic drive (*see* p. 51) which will endeavour to maintain cardiac output and blood pressure to essential organs and will be suggested by the patient's anxiety, tachycardia, and cool, pale, moist skin. Nausea and urine retention may also be manifest. A second compensatory mechanism which will indicate raised pulmonary venous pressures and/or hypoxia is an increase in depth and rate of respiration, especially on exertion. The accessory muscles may be used to aid expansion of the thorax to increase inspiration. A wheeze and cough, with or without sputum, may be present. Systemic hypoxia will cause a central cyanosis and bluish tinge to the face and chest, which is an extremely serious sign. Peripheral cyanosis of lips, nail beds, ear lobes, hands and feet is a sign of low cardiac output.

Other signs of a severely reduced cardiac output and hypotension include oliguria, restlessness and mental confusion. Chest pain may be present, with or without monitor evidence of ST or T wave changes or arrhythmias.

CAUSES

Before considering some of the investigations of left ventricular failure, it is worth outlining the main causes.

1 Very fast tachycardias or heart blocks.

2 The effects of extensive myocardial infarction where a large mass of left ventricular muscle mass has died.

3 The mechanical defects that may follow myocardial infarction, either immediately or after several weeks, e.g. septal defect, ventricular aneurysm, ruptured chordae tendineae or papillary muscle.

4 Valve dysfunction, due to calcification, stenosis, or incompetence, can strain the left ventricle to the extent that it dilates, hypertrophies and becomes ineffective. Active bacterial endocarditis can so severely damage the valves that sudden and severe heart failure can occur, producing shock and circulatory collapse.

5 Restrictive pericarditis can lead to tamponade, where atrial filling is so restricted that cardiac output falls. Trauma, cardiac surgery, and tubercular or malignant effusions can cause tamponade.

6 Toxins from septicaemia or direct infection of the myocardium can mimic myocardial infarction.

7 A massive pulmonary embolism will cause central cyanosis, raised CVP, and circulatory collapse.

8 A dissecting or leaking aortic aneurysm will produce pain, hypotension, possibly myocardial infarction and circulatory collapse.

INVESTIGATIONS

A number of immediate investigations should be performed to fully assess the patient's condition. These include a medical examination, history, and chest X-ray; urgent estimations of serum electrolytes and possibly cardiac enzymes; a blood gas analysis to determine the degree of hypoxia and acidosis; urgent echocardiography, cardiac catheterization, and angiography. The nurse should assist with these procedures to prevent the patient from exertion.

In addition, to aid diagnosis and to monitor progress, the following catheters and lines will be inserted: urine catheter, central venous pressure or Swan – Ganz pulmonary artery line, an arterial line to monitor blood pressure and to facilitate the taking of repeat blood for gas analysis, and finally probes to monitor central and peripheral temperature.

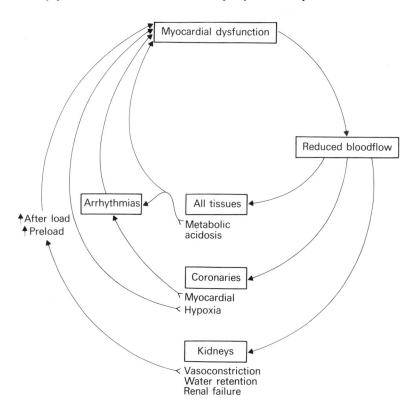

Fig. 5.1   The vicious cycle of cardiogenic shock.

Potential problems and treatment of cardiogenic shock

One of the presentations of acute heart failure is cardiogenic shock. This occurs because the vasoconstriction mechanisms to maintain blood pressure are ineffective, and a vicious cycle develops (Fig. 5.1) which leads to almost certain death. Cardiogenic shock is said to exist if blood pressure is less than 12 kPa (85 mmHg) systolic, if the patient is peripherally 'shut down' (skin pale, cool, and sweaty), with urine output minimal (oliguria) or absent (anuria) and possible mental confusion. However, there is a normal or raised CVP and a near normal heart rate. Note that the shocked state is therefore *not* due to hypovolaemia or arrhythmias.

The low perfusion to the individual organs gives easily recognizable symptoms and signs, which will now be discussed.

LUNGS

The failing left ventricle will become distended and full of blood, the pressures within the ventricles, the left atrium and pulmonary veins will rise. The patient will be extremely breathless. The interstitial lung spaces will become full of oedema fluid, gaseous exchange will be impaired producing poor oxygenation of arterial blood. Hypoxia will further impair contractility of cardiac muscles, and will increase tissue hypoxia and acidosis.

The water-logged lungs will be stiffer to expand, so increasing energy requirements and heart work. A potent diuretic (e.g. frusemide 80 – 250 mg i.v.) will be given to promote excretion of salt and water from the circulation and so reduce interstitial lung water and preload. Diamorphine i.v. 5 mg will reduce anxiety, respiratory drive, and afterload.

The nurse can help by positioning the patient in a head-up position, resting comfortably on pillows. Ensure that the oxygen mask or nasal cannulae are fitted comfortably. Discourage the patient from talking or coughing too frequently, as these will increase hypoxia and necessitate removal of the oxygen mask.

If the patient becomes hypoxic, or the work of breathing excessive, positive pressure ventilation may be instituted. The patient should be sedated and given repeated reassurance and explanations when ventilated. Paralysing agents may be necessary to stop the patient fighting the ventilator but diamorphine, papaveretum or phenoperidine *must* also be given, in spite of hypotension, to allay anxiety and to decrease sympathetic stimulation.

MYOCARDIUM

Low perfusion through the coronary arteries will produce myocardial ischaemia and acidosis, this will impair contractility further with the risk of arrhythmias, heart blocks, and infarction extension. Cardiac output will fall.

The nurse should encourage the patient to rest to reduce tissue and myocardial oxygen requirements. The patient should be positioned in a head-up position, or however he is most comfortable. Sedatives may be given to encourage rest and sleep. Any exertion should be avoided. The patient should have minimal washing or other disturbances, including noise, interruptions, and visitors. Observe the monitor for any change in rhythm since arrhythmias can increase the heart work and reduce cardiac output. The onset of atrial fibrillation can reduce cardiac output by 30%, which can be catastrophic in the shocked patient.

Sedatives such as i.v. diamorphine will aid the patient to rest and settle, and should also be given for any further cardiac pain in spite of the hypotension. Vasodilators of glyceryl trinitrate, isosorbide or nitroprusside may effectively aid the heart by off-loading it. Cardiac stimulants of adrenaline, dopamine or dobutamine may be given by infusion (*see* pp. 111–12).

KIDNEYS

With a blood pressure of below 90 mmHg systolic, filtration at Bowman's capsule will be reduced or cease, causing oliguria or anuria. If blood pressure is not restored quickly, renal failure from acute tubular necrosis will occur. This in turn will cause the blood urea level to rise, which can alter capillary permeability. Pulmonary oedema will occur or be exacerbated. High potassium, urea, and metabolic acidosis cause myocardial irritability which can produce fatal arrhythmias. Metabolic derangement also impairs contractility.

Low bloodflow to the kidneys triggers a chain reaction via the juxtaglomerular apparatus (*see* pp. 37–8). Fluid retention and vaso-constriction will occur. The consequent increase in preload and afterload will further strain the heart.

The nurse should therefore monitor and record blood pressure and urine output closely. A urine output of less than 30 ml for two consecutive hours may require diuretics to be given, or the infusion of low dose dopamine via an infusion pump to dilate the renal arteries to maintain kidney function. To determine body fluid requirements, a CVP or Swan-Ganz catheter will be inserted (*see* p. 11).

BRAIN

Reduced perfusion, with added hypoxia and raised urea, result in altered conscious states. Restlessness, confusion, irritability, or drowsiness are common in cardiogenic shock. Unconsciousness occurs with extreme hypotension, but the patient should not be nursed head down, as cerebral oedema can occur. The confused and restless patient will thrash about and try to remove his oxygen mask and infusions. Heart work will be increased and vital blood will be used to perfuse the exercising muscles instead of essential organs.

The nurse will need to encourage maximum rest with minimal interference. Simple explanations of procedures and answering the patient's questions frankly will aid even the most confused patients. Restraining the patient will only aggrevate his confusion. If the patient is hypoxic, the nurse needs to persevere, with inexhaustable patience, in his wearing of an oxygen mask or nasal cannulae, whichever the patient tolerates better.

Following any arrest of cardiac output, dexamethazone may be given to reduce any cerebral oedema that may result from hypoxia.

ALIMENTARY TRACT

Visceral blood vessels constrict to conserve cardiac output for vital organs; digestion, absorption, and gut mobility are therefore reduced and nausea, vomiting, and constipation may result. Back pressure from a raised central venous pressure on the liver and portal system cause distension and discomfort.

The nurse should offer small amounts of fluids and only a very light diet. Bowel sounds may cease altogether, so no diet is indicated for a day or two. Anti-emetics should be given, especially if narcotic analgesics are used, and medications may have to be given intravenously since they are not tolerated orally.

Aperients will be needed after two or three days to prevent discomfort and straining at stool, but while the patient is in shock he will be too ill to use a commode. The restriction on fluids and the vomiting require frequent mouth washes and care. In prolonged illness, thrush or mouth ulcers may develop and vaseline applied to the lips will help prevent cracking sores, as will humidifying oxygen.

SKIN

Catecholamine release and low cardiac output cause peripheral shut down. The skin becomes cold, pale, and clammy. Peripheral cyanosis will probably be present. The areas subjected to body pressure will quickly become sore due to poor skin oxygenation. (The anaerobic metabolism will produce lactic acid which will lead to a metabolic acidosis.)

The nurse can test capillary perfusion by pressing the fingertips or nail beds and seeing how quickly the pink colour returns. During shock, the peripheral temperature will be much lower than the central temperature. An increasing peripheral temperature will indicate that cardiac output and bloodflow are improving.

To avoid pressure necrosis, the patient should be nursed on sheepskins under the heels and buttocks, and his position should be gently changed at least two hourly. Tissue necrosis can occur on the earlobes and back of the head in patients who are vasoconstricted and in shock for many hours, especially those who are receiving adrenaline.

The patient's hands and feet will be cold, so woollen socks will increase comfort. Diaphoresis is common in shocked patients, so cotton pyjamas are preferable, these and bed linen may need frequent changing. Despite this, remember that the patient's need for rest is primary and must be balanced against the necessity of any nursing intervention or disturbance.

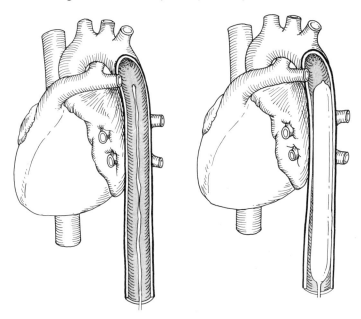

Fig. 5.2 An intra-aortic balloon catheter lying in the thoracic aorta.

Intra-aortic balloon pumping (IABP)

The IABP is a mechanical device to assist the failing heart when conventional drug therapy or emergency surgery are either ineffective or inappropriate. To establish the need for therapy and to monitor its effectiveness the cardiogenic shock patient will require the following: a central venous pressure line (CVP), an arterial line, a Swan – Ganz catheter, a urine catheter, and peripheral and central temperature probes. Oxygen will be administered continuously.

The IABP device consists of a balloon placed in the descending aorta and attached to a bedside console (Fig. 5.2). The balloon is timed by the patient's ECG rhythm to inflate with gas during early diastole and actively deflate before each systole. This simple mechanism assists the heart and body in three main ways: increased coronary perfusion, increased organ and tissue perfusion, and reduction in left ventricular afterload (work). By increasing oxygen available to the myocardium and reducing myocardial oxygen consumption it breaks the vicious cycle of cardiogenic shock.

Increased coronary bloodflow is achieved by the inflating balloon partially blocking the aorta in early diastole, causing some blood to be forced back towards the closed aortic valve and open coronary arteries by a counterpulsation wave. Remember that the coronary arteries are unable to fill during cardiac contraction because the whole myocardium, including the arteries, is squeezed flat. The coronary arteries normally fill during diastole; a raised diastolic blood pressure would therefore greatly increase coronary artery bloodflow, hence improving myocardial oxygenation. The failing heart will receive more oxygen and will pump more effectively and an ischaemic myocardium may be saved from infarction. Arrhythmias induced by myocardial hypoxia and acidosis will be alleviated and no longer impair cardiac output.

Organ and tissue perfusion will be enhanced by the rise in diastolic pressure with the counter pulsation wave, as the balloon inflates. Anaerobic tissue respiration which was producing a systemic acidosis will be reverted by adequate amounts of oxygen reaching the tissues. Bloodflow to the kidneys will increase, so preventing renal failure and promoting diuresis to reduce preload.

The *left ventricular afterload will be reduced* by the active deflation of the balloon just before each systole. The sudden collapse of the balloon in the aorta creates an abnormally low pressure in the root of the aorta enabling the left ventricle to empty itself more thoroughly at systole, the residual volume in the ventricle will fall, so reducing myocardial oxygen consumption (Table 5.1).

INDICATIONS

Because IABP is an invasive device, conventional drug therapy will usually be tried first. If this is not quickly effective, then the vicious cycle of shock begins and an IABP should be inserted.

Apart from cardiogenic shock the balloon can be used for: left ventricular failure (prior to investigation and surgery), congestive heart failure, post-cardiac surgery, rest pain angina (prior to investigation and surgery), left main stem coronary artery stenosis (prior to surgery), and intractable arrhythmias (prior to investigation and surgery).

Table 5.1   When the IABP is inflating and deflating optimally the following can be measured.

Increase in peak diastolic pressure

Decrease in aortic end diastolic pressure

Decrease in pulmonary capillary wedge pressure, with improved blood gas exchange

Decrease in left ventricular end diastolic pressure and preload. CVP lower

Corresponding reduction in left ventricular size — chest X-ray

Increase in pulsatile presssure

Decrease in heart rate

Increase in cardiac output

Decrease in myocardial irritability, i.e. fewer ectopics

Increase in peripheral temperature

Increase in urine output

The patient will improve generally, be less restless or confused Chest pain will resolve, ST changes will settle and the skin will become warmer and dry

---

INSERTION

The balloon is made of polythene in one, two, or three chambers wrapped around a catheter. The insertion method may be a cut down to the femoral artery or the balloon is rolled around the catheter and passed via a cannula into the femoral artery by direct venepuncture. The surgeon will check each femoral artery for a good pulse, and each leg to ensure that even when the balloon is in the artery, the leg will still receive adequate amounts of blood.

The balloon is measured against the patient, and then inserted under local anaesthetic until the tip lies in the descending aorta at the level of the second intercostal space. The level is checked on a chest X-ray.

POSSIBLE COMPLICATIONS

Patient anxiety
Patients who require IABP are invariably already very anxious and distressed about their condition. A doctor will explain to the patient and his family the necessity for this treatment; he will also outline the

procedure of insertion and mechanism of pumping, then obtain a written consent. The nurse invariably has to answer further questions and give reassurance that the operative procedure is small, takes only about 30 minutes, and that the balloon assist is only a temporary mechanism until the heart recovers strength.

Pain and restlessness can occur, for which the patient should be given repeated small intravenous doses of diamorphine and diazepam. An anaesthetist will usually be present to administer these because of the risk of further hypotension. Full intubation and resuscitation equipment should be at hand. The nurse should stay with the patient, hold his hand and explain in simple terms what is happening.

Infection
If the patient is too ill to move to an operating theatre, create as near to theatre conditions as possible in the ward: privacy, no draught, light, space, suction, and diathermy will be required as well as a theatre pack, gowns, and masks. The site is shaved and washed in iodine. Prophylactic antibiotics to prevent local or systemic infection are usually given at the time of insertion and then regularly. A clean, dry dressing should be applied and changed at least twice daily.

Ischaemia of the leg
This may be due to thrombus forming on the balloon in the aorta, thrombus formation in the slower bloodflow in the femoral or iliac arteries, dislodged atheroma, or spasm of the femoral artery around the balloon catheter. To minimize these risks the balloon material is especially designed to reduce platelet stickiness and, prior to insertion, it is rubbed in heparin. The patient will then be given regular heparin.

The patient should not be nursed sitting up higher than a 40° angle, lest occlusion of the femoral artery occurs or the balloon catheter kinks.

The nurse must check both legs hourly for pulse, warmth, colour, sensation, and capillary filling. If at any time she suspects that a leg is becoming ischaemic she should immediately inform the surgeon so that an embolectomy can be carried out. The balloon may need re-inserting in the other femoral artery.

Haemorrhage
This may occur at the site of insertion and cause frank bleeding or a haematoma. However, a pressure dressing should not be used as it may restrict the flow of blood within the femoral artery. Surgical intervention will sometimes be necessary. A small dry dressing should be applied to allow hourly inspection of the area.

Dissection of the aorta

This is an absolute contraindication to balloon insertion. Dissection can be caused at or following balloon insertion, so any complaints of back pain which is not relieved by a postural change should be reported. A chest X-ray may be helpful, and the limb pulses will be carefully checked.

Failure to insert the balloon

Many patients with cardiac disease have disease of the large arteries as well. Atheroma in the femorals, iliacs, or aorta can prevent the surgeon positioning the balloon. In this event, the doctor and nurse should tactfully explain to the patient that, although the balloon assist cannot be used, there are many drugs that are available, but they may take longer to be effective. The patient's family should have the seriousness of the situation explained to them, but the patient must not be allowed to give up all hope as this may itself limit his chance of recovery.

Patient non-compliance

After hours or days the patient may become so restless and feel so restricted by tubes and wires that he will insist on getting out of bed. This can be done if absolutely necessary with *extreme* care not to dislodge the balloon or flex at the hips more than $40°$ which may kink the catheter.

Prop the patient on the edge of the bed or sit him in a chair. Considerable nursing skills are needed to make the patient comfortable in bed for the time (up to three weeks) that the IABP may be in place. Nursing should be grouped to allow rest and sedatives given to encourage sleep. Remove unnecessary restrictions, infusions and monitoring devices as soon as possible. Non-compliance may mean the balloon is removed sooner than is medically desirable to benefit cardiomyopathy, congestive failure or to allow ventricular septal defect, post-myocardial infarction to fibrose sufficiently for surgery.

Balloon dependence

Patients with very poor myocardial function may benefit greatly from balloon pumping, but occasionally it is not possible to wean the patient off the balloon successfully. This is a similar problem to respiratory patients who become ventilator dependent. A medical team discussion including senior nursing staff will decide whether to leave the patient on the balloon for a few more days and to try weaning again, or whether to remove the balloon and allow the patient to develop terminal heart failure. Discussion by all nurses and medical staff helps the patient, his family, and the staff, to cope in the face of failure of medical knowledge to preserve life. Spiritual guidance from the hospital Chaplain or other Minister should be offered to the patient and family at an early stage if appropriate. The staff may also benefit from such help.

The patients who typically become balloon dependent are those who develop severe left ventricular failure and are balloon pumped; they then have angiography in the hope of finding a surgical remedial lesion but are often shown to have extensive myocardial dysfunction. This situation should be clearly explained to the family, but how much the patient will be told will depend on many factors. If the patient should despair of all hope of survival prematurely, this may hinder chance of recovery. Doctors may consider if the patient is suitable for a heart transplantation.

Weaning can begin when benefit from the balloon pump has been achieved (Table 5.2) or the patient has had surgery to correct or bypass any lesion. The balloon pumping may be continued for hours or days following myocardial infarction or left ventricular failure post surgery. Following coronary artery bypasss graft, the balloon will not be necessary unless the ventricular function is poor from previous infarctions.

Explain to the patient that he is progressing well and that the machine support is to be phased out. Reduce the balloon pumping to R wave ratio to 1 : 2. Continue to observe all the parameters for several hours, or overnight. Any sign of deteriorating cardiac output or rise in preload should be reported and pumping ratio increased to 1 : 1 for a further 24 hours. If there is no deterioration, the ratio may be further reduced and/or the balloon volume may be reduced for at least four hours. If the patient remains stable, the balloon will be removed under local anaesthetic with theatre conditions. Bloodflow in the femoral artery will be checked and a Fogarty catheter applied to the artery or repaired if necesary.

After removal of the balloon the patient will require reassurance that his heart can beat effectively without the pump. The nurse should continue to observe the patient's leg pulses and cardiovascular state closely for at least 24 hours. The patient will now be keen and able to get out of bed, especially for toilet purposes. The prophylactic antibiotics and heparin will probably be discontinued. A mobilization programme as for post-myocardial infarction or surgery, whichever is appropriate, can begin.

Delayed wound healing

After removal of the balloon, the wound will be closed with silk and these sutures can be removed after seven days. Several factors delay healing: poor peripheral perfusion, uraemia, and acidosis. If the balloon was *in situ* for several days, it will have acted as a foreign body and irritated the surrounding tissues. The groin site is a difficult area to prepare and keep clean, so local infection is a constant risk. Various dressing methods are used apparently with equal success: dry non-occlusive dressing, dry occlusive dressing, or application of an iodine-containing gel.

Table 5.2   Indications for weaning from the IABP.

Peripheries warm and dry
Urine flow adequate — over 30 ml per hour
Blood pressure adequate — over 13 kPa (95 mmHg)
Return to full mental alertness
Preload reduced to desired level (CVP or PACWP)
Angina ceased, ST segments isoelectric
Heart size reduced on chest X-ray
Lung fields clear of oedema
Arterial blood gases improved, not acidotic, hypoxic or hypercapnic
Any peripheral oedema clearing

MAINTENANCE OF THE IABP

This will depend on the make and model, and a handbook should be kept with each console. However some general points are common to all types.

Gas
The cylinder of helium or carbon dioxide in the console will require changing about every 36 hours. The nurse should find out how to change it and ensure that a spare cylinder is at hand.

Power
The console can run on batteries for one hour only to cover failure or transport. Make sure the batteries are always fully charged. In the event of total balloon console failure, inflate and deflate the balloon manually with a 50 ml syringe a few times every 10 minutes to prevent platelets aggregating on the balloon surface. During this time the patient's cardiac state is maintained with drugs, if possible.

Leaks
Observe for low pressure in the system — some models will sound an alarm, others will visibly pump less effectively. Re-fill the balloon

according to the handbook and, if leaking persists, check the catheter or connecting tube for cracks or kinks. These can be taped or repaired unless the leak is very near the insertion site, in which case the balloon may need to be replaced. Rarely the balloon may rupture; the gas pressure will fall, the augmentation wave will be lost, and blood may be visible in the connecting tube. *Stop pumping* — replacement of the balloon is required.

Re-filling

Several models have an automatic re-filling system but, following alarms or when the rhythm is irregular and the console unable to run on automatic, the balloon has to be filled manually. This simply involves pressing a series of buttons as described in the handbook.

TIMING

The R wave of the ECG informs the balloon console when to inflate and deflate. The nurse's role is to ensure the balloon pump console 'sees' each electrical systole, the QRS. Ensure the ECG trace is clear and free from electrical interference or artifact on minor movements. Place the ECG electrodes to produce a tall positive wave, minimizing all other waves — this may involve some trial and error. If the patient is atrially paced the console can be triggered by the arterial trace.

If the patient is ventrically paced, the pacing spike can be allowed to trigger, but the QRS complex must be smaller than the spike or double triggering will result, rendering the balloon pump ineffective.

On many models the arterial line trace can be used to trigger. The balloon pump expects all rhythms to be almost regular. In atrial fibrillation or if rapid rates occur, the balloon is much less effective. Pacing or more vigorous treatment of arrhythmias than usual may be necessary to produce optimum balloon efficiency.

The ECG is used to trigger the balloon pump, but the timing of inflation and deflation is regulated according to the arterial trace. Fig. 5.3 shows a normal arterial wave form.

1 The aortic valve opens. Point 1 is the aortic end diastolic pressure and marks the end of diastole and the beginning of systole.

2 Peak systolic pressure. Point 2 is the maximum pressure generated by the contracting ventricle. The systolic run-off phase occurs between points 2 and 3; this represents 25% of the stroke volume or cardiac output.

3 Point 3 indicates where the aortic valve closes and diastole begins. When the pressure in the aorta exceeds the left ventricular pressure, the aortic valve closes. The closing of the aortic valve signifies the end of systole and the start of diastole.

To achieve proper timing, the balloon should start to inflate approximately 40 milliseconds prior to the closing of the aortic valve, signified by the dicrotic notch when using the radial arterial line. Approximately 90% of coronary perfusion takes place during diastole. Full balloon deflation is set to occur during aortic end diastolic pressure, or specifically during isovolumetric contraction, because this is the period when the ventricle is generating pressure. Fig. 5.4 shows a 1 : 2 ratio arterial trace of balloon assist.

1 This is the aortic valve opening signifying the end of diastole and the start of systole.

2 This is the peak systolic pressure — the maximum pressure generated by the heart when the aortic valve is opened.

3 This is the peak diastolic pressure. This is the maximum pressure generated by the inflating balloon in the aorta. It is referred to as diastolic augmentation.

4 This represents balloon aortic end diastolic pressure. This is the lowest pressure in the aorta produced by the deflating balloon.

5 This is assisted systole. This point should be lower than point 2, the unaugmented systole.

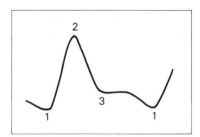

Fig. 5.3 A normal arterial wave form.

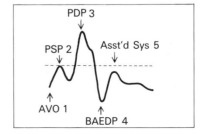

Fig. 5.4 The arterial wave form when the ballon assist is on a 1:2 ratio.

Possible complications of mistiming

If inflation is too early, premature closure of the aortic valve occurs. This produces a decrease in cardiac output and an increase in intraventricular pressures and volume.

If inflation is too late, a reduction in peak coronary perfusion occurs.

If deflation is too early, retrograde flow may occur in the coronary arteries and in other organs. Less than ideal reduction in afterload may also be present.

If deflation is too late, afterload may be increased, This may result in increased left ventricular wall tension and increased oxygen demands upon an already ischaemic myocardium.

IABP case study

Mr James, a 50-year-old man, was admitted to hospital with severe central chest pain. Nine months previously he had suffered a myocardial infarction, since then he had experienced angina on effort. A 12 lead ECG confirmed injury in the inferior leads — ST elevation in leads II, III & AVF. Three hours later Mr James developed complete heart block with a rate of 40 and hypotension. An intravenous infusion of 5% dextrose was commenced and a temporary transvenous pacemaker was inserted after he had been given i.v. atropine 0.6 mg and diamorphine 2.5 mg.

Mr James initially improved, but in spite of a paced rhythm of 90 – 100 beats/minute, his blood pressure fell to 80 mmHg systolic. He was cold, clammy, restless and had not passed any urine. A urine catheter was inserted to monitor urine flow, but he was anuric. A Swan – Ganz catheter was inserted to monitor central venous and pulmonary artery capillary wedge pressures (CVP & PACWP). These were both high (CVP + 14, PACWP 26 mmHg), indicating that shock was definitely not due to hypovolaemia. A radial arterial line was inserted to clearly observe blood pressure.

The IABP was decided on as a cardiac support. Both Mr and Mrs James were seen by a doctor who explained the proposed treatment and a written consent form was willingly signed. The area over both femoral arteries was shaved, he was fasted, placed on a theatre canvas, had rings taped, false teeth removed and was taken immediately to theatre.

Under the local anaesthetic of 1% lignocaine and i.v. sedation of 1 mg diamorphine, a cut down over the right femoral artery was performed and a 40 cm balloon catheter was inserted into the femoral artery and passed into the descending aorta, just below the arch. The balloon console was prepared by a technician, and pumping commenced as soon as the balloon was in place, before the femoral artery and skin were carefully closed over the balloon catheter. Inflation and deflation were set according to the arterial trace to obtain maximal augmentation and presystolic dip.

On return to the ward Mr James was placed on sheepskins and nursed with his head up and resting on several pillows; he was not allowed to flex his right leg more than 40°. Leg perfusion and pulses were checked and recorded. Intravenous heparin and antibiotics were given six hourly. Mr James improved rapidly over the following hours. He was well perfused, with warm, dry peripheries and an adequate urine output. His systolic blood pressure rose to 90 mmHg and PACWP fell to 18 mmHg. Because of his sustained improvement, angiography was carried out, no immediately surgically repairable lesions were seen, only severe coronary artery disease with extremely poor left ventricular function. Improvement continued over the next week: he was sitting up in bed in the ward, talking cheerfully to Mrs James and to other patients, eating a normal diet and requiring only a mild sedative to sleep at night. He was receiving nursing care as appropriate to a patient with recent myocardial infarction on bed rest, with hourly observation of his cardiovascular status, plus leg checks. His ECG reverted to sinus rhythm after two days, so pacing was discontinued.

After six days of IABP therapy, weaning was being considered. Mr James suddenly complained of pain in his lower lumbar region radiating down to both legs. His leg pulses became absent and he was unable to move or feel sensation on his legs. The doctor was notified immediately, and a diagnosis of occlusion of both femoral arteries was made. Diamorphine 5 mg i.v. was given, the situation explained to the patient, and a consent obtained for bilateral embolectomy and balloon removal.

The patient was immediately taken to the theatre where, under local anaesthetic, a saddle embolus across both iliac arteries was removed by Fogarty catheter. The balloon was removed and the femoral artery patched. Good distal bloodflow was achieved to both legs. On return to the ward, both legs were warmer with good pedal pulses; Mr James could feel and move his legs, much to his and our relief.

Mr James had thus survived one of the major complications of IABP in the most severe form. If bloodflow to a limb stops, then gangrene occurs and will necessitate amputation if embolectomy is unsuccessful. Following sudden withdrawal of his cardiac support Mr James's blood pressure fell slightly, but it was 100/70 after three hours and his urine output and perfusion remained adequate. Mr James was a little worried about the loss of his cardiac support, but with the relief concerning his feeling in his legs and much reassurance about his general condition, he overcame his anxiety.

After a further 24 hours of close observations of his cardiovascular state and urine output, his urine catheter, Swan – Ganz line, and arterial line were all removed. A long convalescence of two months was necessary before Mr James returned for coronary artery bypass surgery to prevent further infarction and to enable him to lead a fuller life without angina or breathlessness.

CARDIAC ARREST

The seriously ill patient is obviously at risk, but fit looking patients with cardiac or renal disease may also arrest. There are two main causes: **1** cardiac muscle dysfunction (due to infarction, hypoxia, acidosis, drugs, electrolyte imbalance, arrhythmias, cardiac trauma, electrocution or reaction to radio-opaque dye injection) and **2** inadequate filling or emptying of the heart (due to hypovolaemia, pulmonary embolism, or heart valve obstruction).

Recognition that an arrest of circulation has occurred is straight-forward: a previously conscious patient collapses and will be unrousable, his breathing will initially be in gasps, then stop, the carotid pulse will be absent and the pupils will begin to dilate. An arrest in an unconscious or sleeping patient will be noticed by a change in or by gasps of respiration and a short epileptic-type convulsion that commonly occurs due to cerebral hypoxia.

If the patient is on a cardiac monitor, it will show either ventricular fibrillation or asystole. Prior to the patient losing all cardiac output, the monitor may show ectopics, extreme bradycardias, heart block or tachycardias. Ventricular fibrillation indicates that the heart is extremely irritable; prompt defibrillation can revert the rhythm to sinus and the patient will be none the worse. If nurses are trained and encouraged to defibrillate patients, then sinus rhythm can be restored promptly, before the patient stops breathing, the heart becomes anoxic and acidotic, or irreversible brain damage occurs. If defibrillation is not promptly successful then all heart action will cease and the monitor will show asystole which will require vigorous drug therapy to stimulate heart action.

The longer a patient is left without circulation and tissue oxygenation, the less likely he is to recover. Even if there is no one present who can defibrillate the patient or give intravenous drugs, effective external cardiac massage and artificial respiration will maintain circulation and oxygenation until trained personnel and equipment arrive.

Treatment

(A – Airway, B – Breathing, C – Circulation, D – Defibrillation or Drugs)

AIRWAY

Cardiac arrest may be secondary to a respiratory arrest because the airway is blocked. Extending the neck, and lifting the chin and tongue forward may allow the patient to re-start breathing. This manoeuvre is still essential even if the arrest is primarily cardiac.

BREATHING

If breathing does not re-start when the airway is cleared or when a cardiac rhythm returns, then artificial respiration must be established. Mouth-to-mouth respiration is quite adequate if a mask, airway, or ambubag and 100% oxygen are unavailable. A cuffed endotracheal tube should be passed if the patient does not resume breathing.

CIRCULATION

If the patient is unconscious and has no carotid pulse, give a firm thump with a clenched fist directly over the heart. This may revert ventricular fibrillation or asystole if carried out promptly. Check the pulse (or the monitor) and, if there is not rhythm, summon help and commence cardiac massage.

External cardiac massage

Circulation can be re-started and maintained by squeezing the heart between the sternum and the vertebrae about 60 times a minute. The patient should be lying flat on a firm surface (either the floor or preferably on a bed with a board under the back or under the mattress. A tea tray can be placed across the bed under a child). If the patient is on the floor, kneel beside him; if he is in bed and you are not tall, stand on a stool or kneel on the bed. Place your hands one on top of the other, and place the heel of the lower hand over the lower third of the patient's sternum (Fig. 5.5).

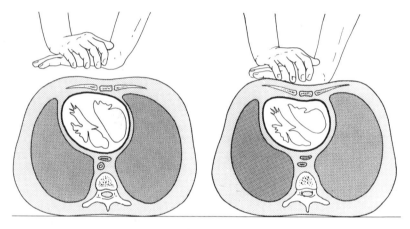

Fig. 5.5   The position of the hands for external cardiac massage.

Men have to be cautioned not to use too much strength or rib fractures can occur; however, to effectively depress the sternum the necessary 1½ – 2 inches (4 – 5 cm) in an adult requires some strength and can be ineffective and exhausting unless a continuous rhythm of compression and relaxation is established. In an infant, the compression must be performed with two fingers only.

This rhythm need not be broken to oxygenate the lungs. Artificial respiration can be given gently without interrupting massage but, if this is too difficult, stop massage briefly after each six compressions to inflate the lungs.

If you are in the unlikely situation of being alone with the patient for many minutes, put oxygen tubing in the patient's mouth (extend the airway) and enough gas will diffuse in and out of the lungs with the movement of cardiac massage.

If the massage is effective it will produce a palpable femoral pulse, and the pupils will be reactive or small.

DEFIBRILLATION

This is the delivery of an electric shock through the heart. It is the only treatment for ventricular fibrillation (VF) because it depolarizes all the heart tissue at one time, regardless of the state of polarization of individual myocardial cells. The sinus node is the quickest tissue to re-polarize, hence sinus rhythm can be restored. Defibrillation also effectively reverts tachycardias and atrial fibrillation. However, the shock causes unpleasant muscle spasm and some myocardial damage, so it is only used on the unconscious patient in an emergency or for non-emergency cases where drug therapy is ineffective where the patient will be anaesthetized first (*see below*).

The nurse should feel for a carotid pulse immediately VF is suspected. If none is present, screen and lie the patient flat. Then charge the machine to 200 – 400 joules and apply small amounts of jelly, or pre-jelled pads, to the right anterior chest wall and left chest, under the axilla (Fig. 5.6). Too much jelly can cause the shock to track across the skin, not through the heart, causing skin burns and an electric flash — but no rhythm change. Place the paddles firmly over the pads or jelly, and, before pressing the discharge button, call for all staff to stand clear of the bed, and do so yourself or you might receive a shock. Discharge the defibrillator. Check the pulses and monitor for resumption of a rhythm and, if defibrillation has not been successful, repeat the procedure with a higher charge. If this is still not effective commence cardiac massage, artificial respiration, and insert an i.v. line and administer drugs to treat the cause of VF as detailed below.

If the VF becomes a very fine or wavy trace, the ventricles should be stimulated with i.v. adrenaline, calcium or even digoxin prior to the next shock.

If VF is persistent, treat acidosis (*see below*), hypokalaemia with i.v. potassium, hyperkalaemia with i.v. glucose plus insulin, and digoxin toxicity with i.v. phenytoin sodium.

When a rhythm is restored, anti-arrhythmic drugs, e.g. i.v. lignocaine, should be given to prevent a recurrence.

Elective cardioversion

This is used for tachycardias, atrial flutter, or fibrillation, and is essentially the same as emergency defibrillation except that the patient will be conscious, the charge is smaller, and VF can be precipitated if the shock should fall on the vulnerable period of the cardiac cycle (T wave). To avoid this, the shock is synchronized to fall within the QRS complex; this is achieved by connecting the patient's monitor to the defibrillator and using its synchronized mode.

The procedure should be carried out in an anaesthetic room or similarly equipped private area. The patient should be prepared as for angiography including fasting and consent and given a short-acting anaesthetic. Intubation equipment should be ready for use, but an airway and oxygen mask are usually sufficient.

In longstanding atrial fibrillation, clot may have formed in the atria; this could embolize after cardioversion when the atria contract properly. Anticoagulants will therefore be given for several days prior to elective cardioversion. Digoxin therapy will be stopped for at least 24 hours prior to cardioversion as fatal arrhythmias may be caused.

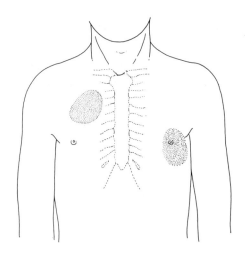

Fig. 5.6   Position of electrodes for defibrillation.

Complications
Following the procedure the patient should be closely observed even if none of the problems outlined in Table 5.3 have occurred.

Table 5.3   Possible complications of cardioversion.

If patient not in VF, this may be caused

Staff electrocution by patient or bed-contact, possibly also causing VF

Burn marks to chest wall due to too much gel being used and DC current tracking across the chest. Pads overcome this problem

Pain from sudden muscular contraction

Distress to other patients

Pain and distress to a conscious patient

Failure of rhythm to revert

DRUGS

A number of drugs are used in the treatment of cardiac arrest; they are summarized in Table 5.4.

Table 5.4   Drugs used in cardiac arrest.

Indication	Drug used
Acidosis	Sodium bicarbonate
Asystole	Chronotropic and inotropic agents
Poor contractility	Inotropic agents
Irritability	Anti-arrhythmics
Electrolyte imbalance	Potassium or glucose + insulin
Digoxin toxicity	Phenytoin sodium

Patient problems

ACIDOSIS

Cardiopulmonary arrest will result in a metabolic and respiratory acidosis. The acidotic heart will be very irritable and contract poorly; ventricular fibrillation and asystole will resist treatment.

Patients who are quickly defibrillated and who have not stopped breathing may not require bicarbonate, but all other arrested patients will;

the amount will depend on the length of the arrest and the size of the patient. Approximately 1 mmol/kg should be transfused rapidly initially, then half that amount given every 10 – 15 minutes if the arrest continues. Sodium bicarbonate 8.4% has 1 mmol/ml so 50 – 100 ml will be given to an adult. Too much bicarbonate will produce an alkalosis, causing a depression of respiration. If bicarbonate 'tissues', tissue necrosis will occur, it should therefore be given via a central vein if possible.

ASYSTOLE, POOR CONTRACTILITY AND BRADYCARDIA

Atropine 0.6 – 1.2 mg i.v. will effectively speed bradycardias; if this is given as soon as a severe bradycardia is noticed on the monitor, asystole may be averted. Atropine increases sinus node rate and AV node conduction, but it does not cause ventricular irritability.

Adrenaline 1 : 10 000 1 – 10 ml i.v. or 1 : 1000 10 – 40 ml in an infusion, has a strong chronotropic and inotropic action. It increases heart rate, AV conduction, myocardial irritability and contractility; if too much is given the patient will develop a tachycardia and possibly ventricular fibrillation. Adrenaline also causes vasoconstriction and so raises the blood pressure.

Isoprenaline 200 μg i.v. or 5 mg in 500 ml infusion has a similar action to adrenaline, but it causes less vasoconstriction.

Calcium chloride 5 mmol i.v. has a strong inotropic effect. It stimulates the heart to start contracting from asystole, and will strengthen the contractility of an already beating heart; however, in the latter case it should be given more slowly or it may cause bradycardia and asystole. Calcium should not be given in the same i.v. line as bicarbonate or precipitation will occur.

IRRITABILITY (*see also* arrhythmias)

This may have caused the arrest, or other arrhythmias may occur after the arrest has been reversed.

A lignocaine bolus of 50 – 100 mg will revert ventricular tachycardia and should then be given as an infusion to prevent the recurrence of either the tachycardia or ventricular fibrillation.

Other anti-arrhythmic drugs include disopyramide, verapamil, mexiletine, bretylium, and beta blocking agents.

Patient care after cardiac arrest

Emotive expressions such as 'Your heart stopped, but we managed to start it again' should be avoided. Telling the patient he collapsed with a serious but temporary disorder of his heart rhythm is true but probably less dramatic or alarming. The relatives, and possibly a Minister of religion, must be informed either by the senior nurse or doctor — preferably someone who has had previous contact with the family — of what has occurred and what the treatment is now to be. The patient may be moved to a coronary unit if not already in one, he will be observed closely for heart rhythm and signs that the temporary lack of cardiac output did not cause cardiac, cerebral, or renal damage. Dexamethazone 5 – 10 mg will be given to reduce any hypoxic cerebral oedema in patients who fail to regain consciousness quickly.

A 12 lead ECG and chest X-ray will be taken to detect the cause of the arrest, and to see if any damage to ribs has occurred during cardiac massage. Pneumothorax or inhalation of vomit could also have occurred. Blood samples for blood oxygenation, acidity, and electrolytes will be taken and levels corrected as necessary.

The patient can be nursed sitting in a comfortable position, and should be treated and observed by the nurses as for myocardial infarction with pain and anxiety relief with diamorphine, monitoring, intravenous cannula, and oxygen therapy. Artificial ventilation may occasionally have to continue for a few hours or days, the heart having been re-started successfully, but not until the brain and respiratory centre had been damaged either temporarily or permanently.

Table 5.5   Cardiac arrest procedure.

Action	Rationale
Establish arrest has occurred, feel for carotid pulse	Radial pulse may not be felt in hypotensive or vasovagal faints.
Ensure airway is patent, remove false teeth and extend the neck.	Breathing may re-start spontaneously, if obstruction was the cause of respiratory arrest. Air and oxygen can diffuse in and out of lungs with the force of cardiac massage alone
Lie the patient flat on firm surface (bed with under-bed board or floor). Use tray under shoulders for children	Cardiac massage will be ineffective on a springy bed
Precardial thump over heart with clenched fist	Shock of thump may revert VF and re-start the heart. Take care not to fracture the ribs

Table 5.5 (cont.)

Action	Rationale
Commence cardiac massage — heel of hands over mid-sternum. Compress sternum 2 inches (5 cm) towards spine then relax; repeat about 60 times/minute (*See* Fig. 5.5)	Re-establish circulation quickly to prevent brain damage. Heart may re-start with flow of blood to coronaries. For babies use two fingers or thumb only; for children one hand will be sufficient
Summon help. The second nurse can start ventilation if still absent (mouth to mouth or airway, mask, Ambu bag with oxygen when available).	Other nurses call team of doctors, collect equipment, screen other patients. Expired air still contains 16% oxygen so mouth to mouth adequate until equipment available; but Brook two-way airway more acceptable and effective.
Attach patient to monitor	Observe: is cardiac arrest due to a slow or absent rhythm, or VF? What are effects of treatment?
If there is ventricular fibrillation (VF) defibrillate patient with 200 – 400 J if trained to do this and ward policy allows; otherwise prepare for use	VF is a common cause of cardiac arrest and can only be terminated by defibrillation. The sooner it is carried out the higher the chance of success
Prepare intubation equipment, assist anaesthetist with suction and oxygen	Restoration of oxygenation as soon as possible with the airway protected by cuffed tube to prevent aspiration of vomit. Oxygenation should be possible without disturbing cardiac massage and circulation of blood
Prepare intravenous equipment, Assist setting up of i.v. infusion (jugular veins often used)	i.v. line needed to give drugs. Neck veins distended in circulatory arrest and easy to cannulate
Give sodium bicarbonate 8.4% 50 – 100 ml i.v.	To reverse respiratory and metabolic acidosis. Acidosis impairs myocardial contractility and causes irritability. Too much bicarbonate will cause an alkalosis, making the patient reluctant to breathe
Continue cardiac massage until rhythm and circulation restored or medical team decide to stop resuscitating	Continuous circulation necessary to deliver oxygen and any drugs given to heart and tissues

Chapter 6
Specific heart diseases

VALVE DISEASE

Besides rheumatic fever, heart valves may become ineffective due to congenital malformation or to disease of their supporting valve rings or chordae tendineae.

Congenital malformation is rare but the aortic valve may have two not three cusps which will cause it to become incompetent in later life. Papillary muscles and chordae tendineae may rupture due to disease or trauma, which will immediately render the atrioventricular valves ineffective. Heart valves may have their annulus stretched out of shape by the failing dilated heart which will make them incompetent and heart failure worse.

Rheumatic heart disease

Rheumatic heart disease fortunately does not affect so many people today as formerly due to better housing conditions and better general health, plus the early detection and treatment of the haemolytic streptococcal sore throat or scarlet fever that may precipitate rheumatic fever. Children and young adults are particularly prone to this disease, though it may occur and recur at any age.

SYMPTOMS

The auto-immune reaction to the streptococcus affects connective tissue of the joints, muscles, tendons, heart valves, and blood vessels. Typically joint pains follow 1 – 3 weeks after a sore throat. The synovial membranes become inflamed, hot, and tender, the patient is tachycardic, pyrexial and sweats profusely. In many cases the illness is less severe with malaise, fatigue, weight loss and vague joint aches attributed to growing pains in the child or arthritis in the adult. Rheumatic nodules may appear over bony prominences and irregular or crescent-shaped erythema may come and go over large areas of the trunk. Blood tests show a polymorphonuclear leucocytosis, anaemia, and raised erythrocyte sedimentation rate (ESR).

149

Table 6.1   Valve disease summary.

Defect/aetiology	The patient	Diagnosis	Treatment
Aortic Stenosis Obstruction to bloodflow from LV to aorta. Congenital bicuspid valve. Fused cusps from rheumatic fever, bacterial endocarditis. Calcification of a congenital defect, or of a normal valve in the elderly	Dyspnoea on exertion, PND, angina, dizziness, syncope	*ECG*: shows LV strain *CXR*: normal or pulmonary congestion plus large LV. Calcified valve *Angiography* shows gradient and LV function	Mild: avoid strenuous exercise; review yearly Severe: urgent replacement
Subvalvular stenosis Congenital fibrous diaphragm or fibromuscular ring below normal valve	As above	Similar to valve stenosis	Resection of obstructing tissue
Regurgitation Valve closure incomplete in diastole. Blood flows back to LV from aorta. Rheumatic fever, Marfan's syndrome or syphillis. SBE can cause acute and severe symptoms	Heart failure, dyspnoea, angina, acute pulmonary oedema	*ECG*: mainly normal *CXR*: pulmonary congestion, heart enlargement *Cine angiography* *Ultrasound*	Control of heart failure. Valve replacement often needed urgently if SBE the cause

Mitral valve stenosis Resistance to bloodflow from LA to LV, raising pulmonary venous pressures. Rheumatic fever, rarely congenital	Lethargy, dyspnoea, haemoptosis, right heart failure, oedema, emboli, chest pain, atrial fibrillation common	*ECG*: large P wave (P mitral) or atrial fibrillation, right heart hypertrophy *CXR*: LA enlarged, pulmonary venous congestion, PA enlarged, ?pul. effusions *Echocardiography*	Treat heart failure, diuretics valve repair, valvotomy, valve replacement
Mitral incompetence Incomplete valve closure at systole. Marfan's syndrome, congenital, ASD, rheumatic fever — ruptured chordae tendineae following MI. Annulus stretched from heart failure	Effort dyspnoea, tiredness, congestive failure	*ECG*: LA + LV enlargement. *CXR*: As stenosis *Echocardiography* *Cine angiography*	Treat heart failure, valve replacement prophylaxis against SBE
Tricuspid valve stenosis Obstructs bloodflow from RA to RV. Rheumatic fever with other valves commonly involved	Fatigue, oedema, hepatic congestion	*ECG*: tall P wave (P pulmonale), atrial fibrillation common *CXR*: large RA Other valve involvement seen *Echocardiography*	Treat congestive failure, diuretics, tricuspid valvotomy or replacement

Table continued over

Table 6.1 (cont.)

Defect aetiology	The patient	Diagnosis	Treatment
Tricuspid incompetence Leakage from RV to RA during systole. Commonly due to dilation of RV from cor pulmonale stretching annulus.	Oedema, hepatic pain, jaundice, ascites; if congenital, cyanosis	*ECG*: WPW syndrome. Bundle branch blocks *CXR*: mild to enormous heart enlargement	Treat heart failure, replace diseased mitral valve, tricuspid replacement or annuloplasty.
Traumatic blunt injury or in road accident, rheumatic fever, congential Ebstein's anomaly			Treat failure, valve replacement

Apart from valve damage, myocarditis with cardiac failure and pericarditis, either dry or with large effusions, can occur. Sydenham's chorea may appear 2 – 6 months after the onset of the sore throat. The neurological symptoms manifest as continuous uncoordinated movements of the hands, face, and feet. These distressing symptoms may occur for up to two years and may recur in pregnancy.

TREATMENT AND RECOVERY

Unfortunately there is no specific medical treatment once the illness has begun and it tends to recur. The joints recover completely but the heart may be irreparably damaged with valve, muscle, and pericardial involvement. Treatment of the acute case includes salicylates for fever, pericardial and joint pain; diuretics for heart failure; and steroids in severe cases. The most important aspect of treatment is *bed rest*. Reduced activity is essential until signs of active cardiac involvement have resolved, as ascertained by reduced fever, weight gain, normal heart rhythm and blood count, with a reduction in the heart size and a return of the ECG to normal. Physical activities can then be gradually introduced as guided by careful monitoring of the sleeping pulse rate to minimize permanent cardiac damage. Convalescence may take months, during which time provision for schooling must be made. To prevent recurrence of the active disease, penicillin is given prophylactically until at least adulthood and possibly for life. Two or more attacks of the active disease make valve damage very likely.

As the active disease process finishes, healing and the fibrosis of the heart valves will involve scarring which will distort and narrow the valves. Therefore follow-up by outpatient visits and a fully informed patient and general practitioner are important. Recognition and control of heart failure with digoxin and diuretics and/or surgical intervention are often necessary. 60% of patients later develop heart disease (commonly mitral valve regurgitation) but some develop a rheumatic cardiomyopathy. Depending of which valves were principally involved by the disease, symptoms of left or congestive cardiac failure may occur. These may be immediate or occur after years of cardiac hypertrophy and other compensatory mechanisms.

ENDOCARDITIS

The heart valves are covered by endothelium and so are very much affected by endocarditis. The inflammation of the endocardium will cause platelets to aggregate on the wall, and vegetations of fibrin, dead cells, and the active bacteria to build up. These vegetations can be seen to flap on echocardiography as the blood flows through the heart and they may break off to embolize.

Acute bacterial endocarditis

This attacks even previously healthy heart valves to cause fever with rigors, profuse sweating, and weight loss. Systemic septic emboli are a real threat, so the disease is treated vigorously with high-dose antibiotics according to blood culture. Staphyloccus, streptococcus, or pneumococcus are usually the responsible organisms — their site of entry to the bloodstream is often obvious following septic abortion, trauma, or other surgical procedure.

Subacute bacterial endocarditis (SBE)

This usually attacks hearts previously diseased either from congenital abnormalities (e.g. patent ductus arteriosus (PDA), bicuspid aortic valve, ventricular septal defects) or valves previously damaged by rheumatic fever. SBE is a subacute, though extremely serious illness and causes malaise, anaemia, anorexia, and extreme weight loss. A persistent low-grade fever is present but blood cultures will not always be positive. The spleen may be enlarged and the kidneys seriously affected to give haematuria, and renal failure from nephritris or microemboli. Micro-emboli also produce diagnostic signs of splinter haemorrhages under the nails and retina.

More serious embolization can occur to damage any organ, including the brain. The organism usually responsible is the non-haemolytic *Streptococcus viridans* which may enter the bloodstream from the mouth, throat, or gums, due to infection or dental treatment, especially dental extraction. For people with congenital heart disease or previous rheumatic fever, prophylactic penicillin is tremendously important to cover dental extraction.

TREATMENT

The course of the disease is prolonged and prior to antibiotics it was always fatal. Even now endocarditis seriously damages the heart valves to cause acute or chronic heart failure. Intravenous antibiotic therapy, plenty of rest, and a nourishing diet for at least six weeks are all necessary. Surgical replacement of the damaged valves, either urgently or at a later date, is often needed. Early recognition and prompt antibiotic therapy increase the chance of a good recovery.

The nurse is involved in observing the patient's general condition, weight, urinalysis, and skin to aid diagnosis; she is also the giver or regulator of the intravenous antibiotics. The prolonged intravenous therapy requires meticulous attention to the intravenous site. Cannula support and slow dilute drug administration are important to avoid excessive phlebitis and pain.

The nursing care needed by these patients (*see* Table 6.2) will be similar to that for most patients with heart failure. These patients, however, are often in the 20 – 50 age group with family, social, and financial responsibilities. The prolonged hospitalisation may strain these relationships, and may also involve a financial burden for housekeeping, baby-sitting and visitors' travelling expenses. In addition to the patient's fatigue, this may cause mental frustration and depression, therefore skilled nursing is necessary to promote the maximum rest·with the minimum of discomfort.

MYOCARDIAL DISEASE

Patients with myocardial disease may present with chest pain, fever, venous congestion, or low cardiac output symptoms. Endocrine, connective tissue or other disorders may cause heart muscle disease. Coronary artery disease can cause the heart to malfunction as a pump when areas of muscle become ischaemic, infarcted, fibrosed or aneurysmal (*see* Chapter 7).

Myocarditis

BACTERIAL MYOCARDITIS

This used to be seen in 25% of patients with diphtheria in which bradycardia, heart failure, and low cardiac output resulted from infection of both the conducting system and the myocardium. The bacteria are treated with antitoxin and penicillin to maintain the patient until the disease passes while general management of congestive cardiac failure, and pacemakers for heart blocks, are given. Permanent heart damage does not result from diphtheria.

Parasitic trypanosomiasis (Chagas' disease)
This disease is transmitted by a South American bed bug. In the acute illness, the parasite multiplies in the cardiac muscle causing fever,

Table 6.2 Nursing care plan for subacute bacterial endocarditis.

Problems	Aim	Plan
Prolonged hospitalization and convalescence, social & financial worries, frustration at inactivity, depression	Removal of concern about social & financial responsibilities; acceptance of temporary restrictions of disease	Discuss illness & treatment. Involve family, friends, business associates and social workers. Rest periods & distractions of TV, radio, reading materials, non-exertional hobbies, occupational therapy
Intravenous therapy for 6 weeks; phlebitis, pain, discomfort, loss of sleep, septicaemia	i.v. infusion not a restriction to sleep or daily activities, no infection or inflammation	Aseptic insertion, dressings & drug administration. Secure and support insertion site & tubing. Slow & dilute administration of antibiotics. Use non-dominant arm if possible. Observe for early signs of inflammation
Anorexia, extreme weight loss, pressure sore risk	Return of appetite, no constipation, weight gain, no pressure sores	Consult dietician. Antiemetics may be required before meals. Appetisers of sherry or stout; light nourishing meals; between meal nourishing fluids; family may bring in favourite foods; care of skin & pressure areas

Anaemia, exhaustion, lethargy	Normal haemoglobin, return of energy	Diet rich in iron. Adequate sleep. Sedatives at night, rest periods during day. Explanation and reassurance
Bedrest complications, DVT, pneumonia	No DVT or pneumonia	Leg exercises; walking to & from bathroom; deep breathing and coughing exercises 2 hourly
Possible complications: systemic emboli, acute heart failure, valve dysfunction	Early recognition as urgent surgery may be needed	Observe skin for petechial haemorrhages. Urinalysis for blood. Weigh daily to observe fluid retention. Heart rate and respirations 4 hourly. Note mental state and any muscle paralysis

tachycardia, and hypotension, followed by congestive failure. The disease may be dormant for 20 years before chronic congestive cardiac failure, heart blocks, and arrhythmias occur. General management of heart failure is all one can offer by way of treatment in the disease, which is responsible for 80% of cardiac failure in South America.

Toxoplasmosis may cause cardiac enlargement in some patients.

VIRAL MYOCARDITIS

The most notorious viral infection is rubella which can cause congenital abnormalities in the fetus. Other viruses may produce changes in the heart structure and impair function, notably poliomyelitis, Coxsackie, and influenza viruses.

Patients may present in the coronary care unit with a provisional diagnosis of myocardial infarction but viral myocarditis is more likely to be the cause of the pain if the patient has a pyrexia on admission and a history of a recent respiratory tract infection. The ECG may show tachycardia and non-specific ST and T wave changes, arrhythmias and conduction defects. Heart failure and pericarditis may develop, but circulatory collapse is rare.

General measures for heart failure with rest, fluid balancing, analgesia, and explanation will be needed. The specific virus is difficult to isolate, but recovery is usually complete.

CARDIOMYOPATHY (MYOCARDIAL DISEASE OF UNKNOWN CAUSE)

Cardiomyopathies are grouped according to the change in structure and function of the myocardium as hypertrophic, congestive, obliterative, or restrictive. Depending on the course the disease takes, patients with cardiomyopathy may present with congestive failure, dyspnoea, chest pain, low cardiac output symptoms, systemic emboli or syncope.

All age groups, including children, are affected by this generalized heart muscle malfunction. Direct causes are not known but some are genetically linked, or aggravated by alcohol, pregnancy, hypertension, viral infection, and auto-immune disorders.

Treatment is aimed at relieving the heart of volume and pressure loads, and other general heart failure measures. Specific treatment is available for only a few types of cardiomyopathy, and the patient may die suddenly or after months or years of chronic congestive failure.

HYPERTROPHIC OBSTRUCTIVE CARDIOMYOPATHY (HOCM)

The patient with HOCM may present with syncope, palpitations, angina pain, and dyspnoea. The symptoms may be confused initially with angina on exertion, because every time the patient develops a tachycardia, or sympathetic tone is increased, the symptoms occur. This is because the heart muscle becomes thickened and stiff so that atrial filling in diastole is resisted. The hypertrophied muscle classically protrudes below the aortic valve, so it obstructs ejection at systole.

Syncope and sudden death can result from arrhythmias or the total obstruction of the aortic valve. Angina occurs because the blood supply may be inadequate for the increased needs of the hypertrophied muscle, and dyspnoea will occur due to raised left ventricular and atrial pressures which prevent free bloodflow from the pulmonary veins. X-ray, ECG, angiography, and echograms will confirm the diagnosis.

Treatment is aimed at reducing the sympathetic tone and preventing tachycardias. Beta adrenergic blocking drugs such as propranolol are given in high doses, and the patient is advised not to take sudden strenuous exercise, e.g. heavy lifting. Resection of the obstructing muscle and valve replacement if an enlarged papillary muscle has distorted the mitral valve may greatly improve the patient's symptoms.

If atrial fibrillation occurs, the stiff ventricles will be inadequately filled and severe failure may ensue. Dyspnoea and congestive failure will follow left heart failure.

CONGESTIVE CARDIOMYOPATHY

When all possible reversible causes of congestive failure have been ruled out, congestive cardiomyopathy is said to exist. The disease may affect both ventricles to give symptoms of low cardiac output and venous congestion in a few months. The hypertrophy and some local fibrosis will impair conduction, oxygenation, and pumping efficiency of the myocardium.

Treatment is *bed rest* for prolonged periods and is aimed at relieving the symptoms of oedema and dyspnoea. Preventing complications of emboli, pneumonia, and deep vein thrombosis are also very important.

The patient and family should be encouraged towards only short term goals: relief of dyspnoea and oedema, going home, visiting neighbours and family, and returning to only part time or light work. This is because more ambitious plans may be beyond them and they may be disappointed in themselves and dissatisfied with their treatment.

OBLITERATIVE CARDIOMYOPATHY (ENDOMYOCARDIAL FIBROSIS (EMF)
(OR ENDOCARDIAL FIBROELASTOSIS (EFE) IN INFANTS)

This tends to occur in humid and tropical zones. The ventricular cavities become full of fibrous tissue and thrombus. Valve dysfunction and pericardial effusions may develop and scar tissue can infiltrate the myocardium, preventing the heart filling during diastole or contracting properly at systole. The patient will present with a restrictive and congestive failure, causing oedema, low cardiac output, systemic and pulmonary emboli

There is no specific treatment. General management of heart failure should be given.

RESTRICTIVE CARDIOMYOPATHY

This occurs rarely, and may present as a constrictive pericarditis. The endomyocardium becomes infiltrated by fibrous tissue, preventing filling in diastole and ejection at systole. Amyloid disease may be the cause.

Specific diseases of the myocardium are usually secondary to systemic or metabolic illnesses. Most produce a congestive cardiomyopathy (e.g. acromegaly) but some present with the hypertrophic obstructive type (e.g. Friedreich's ataxia). Amyloid causes a restrictive cardiomyopathy, and sarcoidosis may present with failure, arrhythmias, or conduction defects.

The treatment depends on the cause; symptomatic treatment of heart failure, conduction defects or arrhythmias may be required.

PERICARDITIS

Pericarditis may occur due to many causes, including the following: infections — viral, bacterial or tuberculous, malignancy — cancer of lung or breast, radiotherapy to thorax, uraemia, post myocardial infarction or post open heart surgery (Dressler's syndrome), trauma, rheumatic fever, dissecting aneurysm, myxoedema, drugs — hydralazine, practolol, procainamide, and collagen diseases.

Symptoms and signs

An effusion may or may not be present, and constriction can occur acutely or chronically. The patient will complain of pain and symptoms of heart failure. The patient with a *dry pericarditis* will complain of chest pain, which will be similar to the pain of myocardial infarction, but it will be sharp, worse on coughing, swallowing and on respiration, and relieved by leaning forward. The pain rarely radiates to the arms in pericarditis. A pyrexia, cough, or other respiratory symptoms may be present.

Signs on the ECG will be ST elevation, especially in lead II; atrial fibrillation may occur but the heart shadow on X-ray will not change and signs of calcification may be present on the X-ray in chronic diseases. A pericardial friction rub will be heard by stethoscope.

A large *pericardial effusion* can accumulate quickly to cause cardiac tamponade. Tamponade is a life-threatening situation because the heart cavity is prevented from expanding and filling from the veins. Systemic and pulmonary venous pressures will rise, causing ascites and dyspnoea, and cardiac output will fall. Tamponade should be relieved by pericardial aspiration or cardiac arrest may follow. More chronic pericardial effusion may produce the same severe ascites with raised venous pressure, some dyspnoea, and a reduced cardiac output.

INVESTIGATIONS

Effusions can be clearly seen on echocardiograms, the ECG will appear of small voltage, the heart sounds will be muffled and the heart shadows on X-ray will enlarge — all due to the surrounding fluid. A pericardial frictional rub will still, however, be heard.

Pericardial fibrosis may occur either after an effusion or by itself. The fibrosis may constrict the heart to give a similar picture to a large effusion, but mild constriction may be well tolerated and the resultant failure can be treated medically. Severe or recurrent constriction can be permanently relieved by removing the parietal pericardium at surgery (a pericardectomy.

TREATMENT

The treatment of pericarditis will depend on the cause of the inflammation, but analgesia and relief of anxiety are very important. Mild pain will respond to aspirin or indomethacin, steroids are often effective for more persistent inflammation, especially if it is of auto-immune type, e.g. Dressler's syndrome (post infarction or cardiotomy) or rheumatic fever. Severe pain may require diamorphine for relief.

Venous congestion and ascites may be controlled by diuretics, but severe restriction to venous filling of the heart will necessitate aspiration or pericardectomy.

CONGENITAL HEART DISEASE

Some 8 babies out of every 1000 live births have a congenital heart defect, 13% of these babies have more than one defect and 40% of babies with Down's syndrome (mongolism) also have a cardiac defect. One cause of defects is a rubella infection in the mother during the first three months of fetal growth. A summary of congenital heart diseases is given in Table 6.3 (p. 170).

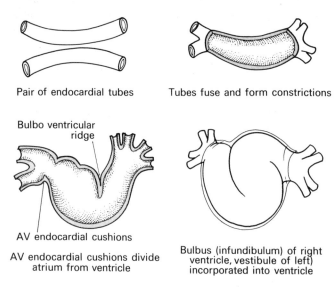

Pair of endocardial tubes   Tubes fuse and form constrictions

Bulbo ventricular ridge

AV endocardial cushions

AV endocardial cushions divide atrium from ventricle

Bulbus (infundibulum) of right ventricle, vestibule of left) incorporated into ventricle

Fig. 6.1   Early development of the heart.

Aetiology

The heart and blood vessels form from two cylindrical tubes of endo-, myo- and epicardium. At the end of four weeks the tubes have twisted together and developed five clear segments of sinus venosus, atria, ventricle, bulbus cordis and truncus arteriosus (Fig. 6.1). The endocardial cushion develops to form the two atrioventricular valves, and sheets of tissue then grow down towards this cushion to form the septum primum (Fig 6.2). The bulbus cordis fuses into the ventricular ridge and, together with the truncus arteriosus, a spiral endocardial cushion develops to divide the aorta and pulmonary artery. The atrial septum primum has a hole in it, called the ostium primum, to allow normal fetal bloodflow. The septum secondum forms, also with a hole which is called the foramen ovale. These two septia form a flap valve so that bloodflow in the fetus can mainly bypass the right ventricle and the non-aerated lungs during intrauterine life to reduce cardiac work. A temporary artery, the ductus arteriosus, allows the passage of all but 5% of the blood that enters the right ventricle and pulmonary artery, to flow directly into the aorta (Fig.6.3). The left and right ventricles will have an equal workload, and will be of equal thickness.

At birth the lungs become aerated and expand. The right heart pressures become less than the left due to the low resistance to bloodflow through the expanding lungs. The atrial flap valve will close and bloodflow through the ductus arteriosus will stop. These closures are usually complete in the first few days of life unless a hypoxic episode causes the ductus to stay open. The right heart muscle will remain thin walled, but the left ventricle will become thicker and stronger to generate enough pressure to overcome systemic arterial pressure.

If a cardiac defect exists, the size and complexity will determine if the infant survives at all, if the infant develops cyanosis and heart failure after a few weeks, or if a defect can be surgically corrected. Many other infants will grow normally and be totally asymptomatic for years, the defect only being suspected when a murmur is heard at a routine medical examination, or heart failure develops in early adult life.

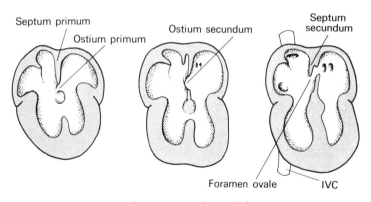

Fig. 6.2 Development of the artrial and ventricular septa.

CYANOSIS

Will occur if the arterial oxygen level falls. If non-oxygenated blood from the right heart or pulmonary artery mixes into the left heart and systemic circulation, e.g. transposition of great vessels (*see* Fig. 6.5) cyanosis will be apparent.

Cyanosis can also occur from non-cardiac lesions. Peripheral cyanosis is common in normal infants for the first few hours of life, and bruising and purpura from the umbilical cord around the neck may at first give the appearance of cyanosis. If the cord is clamped too early the baby may be polycythaemic, the excess of circulating red cells may give the skin a bluish tinge even though the baby is adequately oxygenated. Severe respiratory disorders will obviously give rise to cyanosis, but the chest X-ray should confirm if the cyanosis is due to pneumonia, aspiration of meconium, emphysema, pneumothorax, or a diaphramatic hernia.

Respiratory distress syndrome is more common in premature or Caesarean babies, and in those with diabetic mothers. Neonates breathe

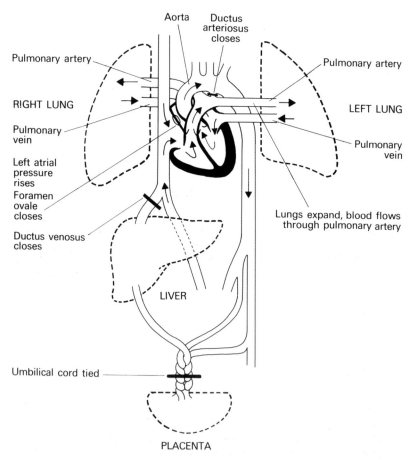

Fig. 6.3 Changes in the fetal circulation at birth.

through their nose and, if choanal atresia is bilateral, severe dyspnoea and cyanosis will develop.

Blood gases taken when the baby is breathing air, and then when the baby is breathing 100% oxygen, should differentiate between a respiratory and a cardiac cause for cyanosis. If the cause is cardiac, where some blood is bypassing the lungs, the oxygenation can only be slightly improved.

Babies with brain damage may have periods of apnoea which will give rise to cyanosis, whereas babies with a cardiac lesion are likely to be dyspnoeic. Cyanosis and dyspnoea will be more apparent on any exertion, especially feeding or crying. The mother may not notice that the baby is dyspnoeic, but complains that the baby is very poor at feeding.

Squatting

Children with Fallot's tetralogy (*see* Fig. 6.4) typically squat after any exertion. This manoeuvre blocks off the femoral arteries so increasing systemic resistance. This increase in pressure will be transmitted back to the left and right ventricles via the septal defect, and will force blood through the narrowed pulmonary artery to increase bloodflow and oxygenation of the lungs.

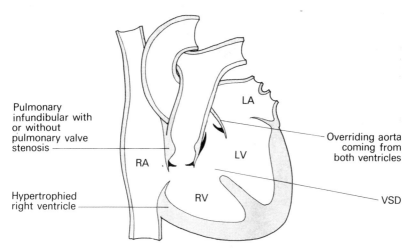

Fig. 6.4 Fallot's tetralogy.

Dyspnoea

Dyspnoea without cyanosis will occur if already oxygenated blood is passing from the left heart back into the right heart to be circulated through the lungs (e.g. septal defects). The volume of blood going through the right heart and lungs will be increased.

This rise in flow and subsequently of pressure within the pulmonary arteries will make the lungs stiff, and will give the chest X-ray the typical signs of plethora. This will lead to interferences in gaseous exchange and recurrent chest infections. Prevention and treatments of chest infections should be vigorous.

An increase in pulmonary vascular resistance and blood volume will cause the right heart to thicken in an effort to eject the extra volume of blood into the pulmonary vessels. In infants, these pulmonary vessels have muscular walls that can reduce the amount of bloodflow to the lungs, and they will constrict in response to acisosis, high CO_2 or low oxygen levels in the blood.

It is therefore important to prevent hypoxia, hypercapnia and acidosis by carefully maintaining a constant inspired oxygen level, and preventing infection by barrier-nursing the baby. Maintaining clear airways and prevention of small airway collapse can be achieved with change of position and active chest physiotherapy.

If pulmonary hypertension develops to such a level that the right heart pressures exceed left heart pressures, the shunt across any defect will reverse to a right-to-left shunt, so bypassing the lungs altogether to give cyanosis and a poor prognosis in these children.

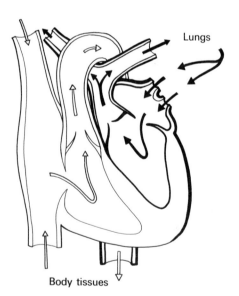

Fig. 6.5 Transposition of the great vessels showing how aorta from the right heart and pulmonary artery from the left heart produce two seperate circuits of oxygenated blood to the lungs and deoxygenated blood to the body.

Heart failure

Heart failure may develop in the first weeks of life, e.g. from pulmonary atresia, or it may not be evident until later in life or old age, e.g. from a small ventricular septal defect (VSD). Either or both ventricles may fail when they can no longer eject all the blood returned to them, because of excessive circulating blood volume or obstruction to bloodflow.

Signs of failure will be apparent: tachypnoea causing difficulty in feeding, tachycardia with rates of 150 – 200/minute, and an enlarged liver. Attention to the baby's weight is important: in the presence of heart failure and fluid retention the baby will not initially lose weight after birth and will then gain more weight than expected for a poor feeder. The baby will have signs of a moist chest and a cough, and may sweat profusely. A large left-to-right shunt produces a poor peripheral bloodflow, but an increased energy output with a high metabolic rate occurs. Sweating may be the only mechanism by which the baby can lose heat to maintain an even temperature.

The earlier heart failure develops, the more serious must be the lesion, even if the baby has no cyanosis or murmurs. If the lesion is operable, then an immediate palliative or complete repair should be carried out — since failure in the first month of life cannot usually be adequately treated medically. Because of the risks of complex cardiac surgery under the age of two years, many surgeons perform palliative procedures to allow the baby to live and grow, then after two years a total correction of the defect will be carried out to prevent further cardiac or pulmonary damage, e.g. Blalock shunt in Fallot's tetralogy. Smaller lesions, e.g. septal defects, are usually repaired before the child reaches school age (*see* Table 6.3 pp. 170 – 4).

INVESTIGATIONS

The physical medical examination will be followed by an ECG, chest X-ray and laboratory blood testing. Cardiac angiography and catheterization will be carried out even in new born infants if it is thought necessary to proceed to surgery.

Where surgery is not immediately necessary or possible, the child will be closely supervised to detect any worsening in heart failure or pulmonary hypertension. Repeat angiography and cardiac catheterization may be necessary before later surgery to correctly identify the haemodynamic effects the lesion has had upon the heart and lungs.

NURSING INTERVENTION

Assessment of the infant's or child's needs will indicate what care to give. Knowledge of care of infants, the specific physiology of the defect, and of the body's compensatory mechanisms is essential. If the infant is well, even though he has a murmur, he is unlikely to become acutely ill, but as in all infants, he will still need careful observation and care against hypothermia, hypoglycaemia, and acidosis.

Nursing care will of course depend on the age of the patient and the degree of disability. Rest is most important. The patient should be allowed periods of uninterrupted rest, with grouping of activities. Crying will demand more energy and cardiac output, so sudden disturbances and noise should be minimized and sedation may be given. Oxygen will almost always be required for a baby with cyanosis or heart failure. Securing the patient in an upright or suspended position may be necessary to minimize the respiratory effort required.

Temperature, heart rate, respiratory rate and pattern, as well as general colour and alertness, should be observed and recorded. Fluid balance and weight charts are also of enormous importance to detect early signs of heart failure. The baby that is quickly investigated and treated, if operable, stands a better chance of survival than a baby that becomes acidotic, malnourished and in severe heart failure. An early accurate diagnosis not only aids the surgeon to decide when and if to operate, but will also allow the medical and nursing staff to frankly and fully discuss the baby's prognosis with the parents.

Parents
The nursing staff not only care for the baby, or child, but the parents and grandparents too. It is important that the nursing, medical, and surgical staff act as a united team, so that a trusting, honest, and caring relationship can be built with the parents. Much information concerning the baby's symptoms will come from the parents: feeding problems, incessant crying, cyanotic attacks, and even syncope. By this stage the parents will be very anxious and tired, and will possibly reproach themselves for some imagined action which they think may be the cause of the baby's illness. Reassurance and encouragement are therefore essential if the parents are to continue handling and feeding the baby, where possible (especially if it is their first). Grandparents, or friends, can greatly help by offering moral support and the experience of their own children.

Mothers are able to stay with or near to their children in many hospitals; however, they may have other children to care for or may become excessively tired and anxious, so that they need a break from the hospital setting.

Mothers, especially of new born babies, should be actively encouraged to assist with feeding and other aspects of care. Some hospitals operate a human milk bank, so that even if the baby is not fed initially, the mother may wish to express her milk to enable her to breast feed at a later date. If the baby is to be tube fed, her milk can be used. This, and the handling of the baby, if only touching him in an incubator, will assist the baby and mother to bond a relationship.

Table 6.3 (pp. 170-4)   Congenital heart disease.

Defect/aetiology	Symptoms	Findings	Treatment
Atrial septal defect (ASD) Failure of septal development. 90% are secundum defects and do not involve AV valves. 5% are sinus venosus defects, these have a high ASD with an anomalous pul. vein	Usually asymptomatic until 30 – 40. Pul. hypertension and heart failure cause progressive fatigue, dyspnoea and haemoptosis. Eisenmenger's syndrome can occur	These will depend on the size and direction of shunt, and the amount of pul. hypertension. Heart failure. *ECG*: Rt. axis, RBBB and first degree block *CXR*: Enlarged atria and pul. vessels. Aorta looks small	Surgical closure on cardiopulmonary bypass, using sutures or a patch of pericardium. Close before school age even if asymptomatic, or close when discovered if older
5% are ostium primum defects of the endocardial cushion. These involve the AV valves and a VSD	Ostium primum defects may cause severe symptoms in infants of failure to thrive, dyspnoea, and repeated chest infections	*ECG*: Lt. axis, atrial arrhythmias	Close ASD and repair valves before school age, or sooner to prevent heart failure and pulmonary problems
Coarctation of the aorta Narrowing of the lumen of the aorta, either before or after the ductus arteriosis. Can lead to dissection of the aorta, bacterial endocarditis, and hypertension. Other defects may be present	Acynotic, but may present in 1st week of life, or not until 20 – 30 years. Symptoms of LV failure, headache, intermittent claudication and tired legs	Hypertension, BP much higher in arms than legs. *ECG*: LV hypertrophy BBB *CXR*: Rib knotching and distorted aortic arch. Upper limbs better developed, collateral arteries visible across chest wall	Resection of narrow portion with an end-to-end anastomosis, or a graft for a longer section. Operate before five years to allow normal growth of lower body. If discovered later an operation will correct hypertension

Eisenmenger's syndrome
Term used to describe cyanotic conditions where the pul. venous pressure = systemic arterial pressures due to high pul. vascular resistance. Any shunt becomes rt. to lt., or bi-directional. Occurs with large ASD, VSD, and PDA, also aorto-pulmonary window, truncus arteriosis, double out-let right ventricle, single ventricle, complete atrioventricular canal.
The large pul. bloodflow increases pul. vascular resistance, but at different rates in individuals

Progressive cyanosis, dyspnoea and fatigue on exertion. Rt. heart failure, haemoptosis and SBE a risk.
Patients usually die by 40 – 50

Cyanosis and clubbing, i.e. nails and tips of fingers and toes are flattened and rounded.
ECG: Rt. axis
P wave tall (P pulmonary)
RV hypertrophy
CXR: Heart size normal
Pul. vessels dilated

Usually inoperable. If shunt has reversed rt. to lt., then an operation is contraindicated because the high pul. vascular resistance needs an escape route, otherwise the pul. hypertension will worsen as will prognosis.
Medical therapy to prevent SBE and thromboemboli.
Chest infection, pregnancy or the contraceptive pill are a real risk

Fallot's tetralogy (see Fig. 6.4)
1   A VSD.
2   Pulmonary infundibular, with or without pul. valve stenosis.
3   Over-riding aorta. The aorta seems to come from both ventricles.
4   Rt. ventricular hypertrophy

May be cyanotic or not, noticed at birth or not until early infancy, depending on size of the various defects.
Infundibular may occasionally close to give cyanotic attacks in which the child goes grey and unconscious.
Squatting may occur after exercise (*see* text)

Progressive cyanosis, effort intolerance and heart failure.
ECG: P wave tall
R wave tall and ST strain in V1 – V3
Rt. axis
CXR: cardiomegaly

Paliative operations to increase pul. bloodflow by bypassing the PA to allow child to live until big enough to survive total correction. Blalock shunt anastomosis of a subclavian artery to a pul. artery. This shunt may block before the total correction at age two.
For cyanotic attacks give urgent therapy to relax pul. outflow tract, i.v. propranolol

Table 6.3 (cont.)

Defect/aetiology	Symptoms	Findings	Treatment
Patent ductus arteriosis (PDA) The ductus is essential for normal fetal bloodflow, but should close soon after birth. It is more likely to stay open if any hypoxic event occurs. Eisenmerger's syndrome can develop	Often asymptomatic until adulthood, then fatigue and dyspnoea on exertion	Toes ONLY may be clubbed. *ECG*: 1° block LV hypertrophy Atrial fibrillation if large lt. to rt. shunt. *CXR*: Large lt. atrium and ascending aorta. PA prominent.	Closed heart surgery, division and tying of ductus before five years, or when discovered, if later
Pulmonary atresia Absent pul. outflow tract. Patent foramen ovalis and PDA essential for survival	Baby is cyanosed and very ill	*ECG*: cardiomegaly Rt. axis RV hypertrophy *CXR*: cardiomegaly and poor pul. bloodflow. Small stature, web neck	Shunts can be made to increase pul. bloodflow
Pulmonary stenosis Narrowing of pul. valve with post-stenotic dilation, or infundibular stenosis. Rt. ventricle hypertophy	Usually asymptomatic and acyanotic in infancy. In adulthood rt. heart failure and chest pains occur. Some people have dyspnoea on exertion and fatigue	*ECG*: Rt. axis RV hypertrophy RA enlarged *CXR*: Large RV Enlarged PA but pul. vasculature normal	Open heart surgery, valvotom to cut fused commissures open Excision of hypertrophied muscle

Transposition of the great vessels Commonest cyanotic lesion in neonates. The aorta and pul. artery arise from the wrong ventricles, therefore two separate circulations exist. The left heart circulates blood through the transposed PA back to the lungs, and the rt. heart pumps deoxygenated blood to the body tissues via the aorta, and back to the rt. atrium. Survival only if the foramen ovalis and ductus remain patent. Other defects of VSD, pul. stenosis may be present	Cyanosed very weak baby. The baby will deteriorate at about one week when the ductus closes. Cyanosis and distress will be marked	*ECG:* not helpful *CXR:* lung markings normal or increased Heart shadow looks like an egg on its side. Baby likely to be large	To increase the mixing of the two circuits so that the baby survives, a Rushkind's septotomy is carried out under angiography. A balloon catheter is passed from the femoral vein to the RA, through the foramen ovalis; the balloon is inflated and the catheter jerked back. A large hole is thus made in the atrial septum. A further corrective operation (Mustard's operation) may be done when the child is two years
Tricuspid atresia Absence of opening between RA and RV, survival depends on foramen ovalis and ductus staying patent	Cyanosis within the first week of life	*CXR:* RV undeveloped. Poor pul. bloodflow Cardiomegaly	A shunt can be made to increase pul. bloodflow

Table 6.3 (cont.)

Defect/aetiology	Symptoms	Findings	Treatment
Ventricular septal defect (VSD) This is the commonest defect. Many VSDs close spontaniously, or get smaller with age. High pul. vascular resistance may persist from birth, or develop in infancy. Pul. hypertension or Eisenmerger's may occur. SBE is a real risk, even after surgical closure. May be associated with aortic insufficiency or pul. outflow stenosis	Small defects will not give symptoms, growth and development normal. Large or multiple small defects may well make a baby ill and in heart failure by six weeks. Child will be frail, of small stature, and have effort intolerance	Small defect — normal ECG and CXR Larger defect — *ECG:* LV hypertrophy Lt. axis *CXR:* LV prominent LA large Main PA enlarged Small aortic knob Heart failure	Leave alone, follow up, give prophylaxis against SBE. Cardiac catheter, if PA pressure ⅔ of systemic pressure, then defect is closed to prevent Eisenmerger's at two years, even if child is asymptomatic. If baby in heart failure, give digoxin and diuretics. If baby too ill or too small for open heart surgery, then PA is banded to reduce pul. bloodflow to stop Eisenmerger's developing. Debanding and closure at age two

Key: ASD = atrial septal defect, AV = atrioventricular, BBB = Bundle branch block, LA = left atrium, LV = left ventricle, PDA = patent ductus arteriosus, PA = pulmonary artery, RA = right atrium, RV = right ventricle, SBE = subacute bacterial endocarditis, VSD = ventricular septal defect

Chapter 7
Coronary artery disease

ANGINA

All tissues require oxygen to function but working muscles will require an increased supply. An increase in cardiac work increases the myocardial oxygen requirements but, if the coronaries are narrowed and the bloodflow reduced, this greater oxygen demand cannot be met and myocardial ischaemia with the pain of angina occurs. This pain mechanism is similar to a stitch from exercising after a meal. To relieve pain the person stops exercising, blood flows to the gut instead of exercising muscles and pain is relieved. In an angina attack the pain forces the person to stop and rest, the heart will thus have a smaller output demanded of it so the myocardium will require less oxygen; this amount can be supplied even by quite diseased coronary arteries. To prevent angina and infarction, a reduction in cardiac workload and consequent oxygen consumption is essential.

OXYGEN AVAILABILITY

Where possible, an artery leading to ischaemic tissue will dilate in an effort to deliver more oxygen. The tissues will extract as much oxygen from the blood as they need. The myocardium extracts more oxygen from its arterial bloodflow than does other body tissue, as can be measured by taking arterial, coronary sinus, and venous blood samples. In health arterial blood contains 19 ml of oxygen per 100 ml of blood if the haemoglobin is 14.5 g/dl. Venous blood will still contain 14 ml oxygen because the tissues have only taken up 5 ml of oxygen per 100 ml of blood. The blood in the coronary sinus, into which the coronary veins drain, contains only 4 ml oxygen, showing that the myocardium has extracted 15 ml of oxygen from the 19 ml available per 100 ml of blood. This leaves little reserve should the arterial blood not be fully oxygenated, the bloodflow restricted, or myocardial oxygen consumption increase.

People with severe anaemia (less than 5 g/dl) will experience angina and heart failure even though the coronary arteries are normal. Those with severe lung disease resulting in low arterial oxygen levels will also have heart failure and angina though their coronary arteries are normal.

OXYGEN CONSUMPTION

This is increased whenever heart work is increased. An obvious example is exercise when not only will contractility increase but so will heart rate. The coronary arteries fill during diastole and are squeezed flat during systole. In fast heart rates (e.g. due to sympathetic stimulation or catecholamine release, exercise, pain, emotion or from abnormal tachycardias), diastole is shortened so that a mismatch of oxygen supply and demand exists. The heart has to work harder to produce the larger stroke volume that is necessary to maintain cardiac output in the presence of extreme or inappropriate bradycardias. Bradycardias and heart failure will also increase the end diastolic pressure within the ventricles. This raised pressure stretches the endocardium so squeezing the coronary arteries to this area and reducing the endocardial supply.

Arterial vasoconstriction demands that the myocardium contracts more forcibly to eject blood into the aorta. This increase in afterload also increases heart work and oxygen consumption.

The coronary arteries

The myocardium is supplied with blood by the left and right coronary arteries (Fig. 7.1). These leave the aorta directly behind the aortic valve cusps and then circle the outside of the heart like a coronet.

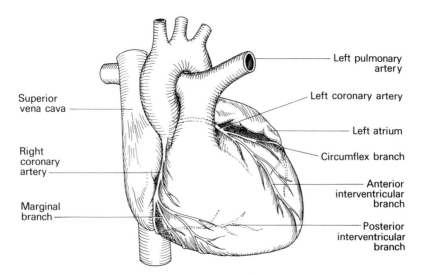

Fig. 7.1 The coronary arteries.

The right coronary artery supplies blood to the myocardium of the atria, right ventricle and the inferior of the left ventricle. A branch of the right coronary artery supplies the AV node.

The left coronary artery soon divides to form the circumflex, left anterior descending, and marginal coronary arteries. These vessels supply blood to the left ventricle and septum. A collateral circulation exists to some extent between the left and right coronaries, particularly between the right coronary and the left anterior descending artery.

The myocardial blood then flows into the coronary sinus in the right atrium.

ATHEROMA

The narrowing of diseased coronary arteries is due to the laying down of atheroma beneath the tunica intima (Fig. 7.2). These plaques are likely to form at bifications where the turbulent bloodflow damages the artery wall allowing the atheroma to start. This then causes roughening of the artery wall, so that platelets stick to the plaque, narrowing the lining of the artery further. The atheroma may then calcify or haemorrhage into itself causing it to swell or the plaque to break away to lodge and block a smaller coronary artery. The atheroma is made of fats (lipids), fibrin, cholesterol and calcium. What actually causes atheroma to occur is not fully understood, but there are several known risk factors associated with atheroma build up.

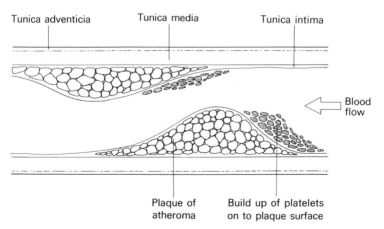

Fig. 7.2   Diagram to show build-up of atheroma in an artery. Note narrowing of lumen, lifting of tunica intima, and platelet build-up.

CAD risk factors

Table 7.1 clearly shows some of the risk factors for developing coronary artery disease. These are discussed more fully below together with the beneficial effects of medication and alteration of lifestyle. However, it is unfortunately all too often the case that the patient may be very reluctant to change his habits or lifestyle, possibly due to denial of his illness. In addition, the patient may not fully appreciate the severity of his illness or be aware or believe that changing his lifestyle for the better can help. Finally, it is possible that he may not know how to change, and in this respect the nurse should take advantage of the good motivation to improve health that follows recent illness to educate the patient and his family about the medical problems and how they can improve the outcome.

Table 7.1   CAD risk factors. Data from the Health Education Council.

Factor	Incidence times normal	
	Women	Men
Smoking	3 – 6	3 – 6
Diabetes	6	6
Hypertension blood pressure increases with age, even mild increases significant. For every 10 mmHg:	1.2	1.4
High cholesterol greater than 280 mg/100 ml	–	4
Age increases steadily with age		
below 60	1	6 (× women)
above 60	high	high
Contraceptive pill previous family history + smoking 20/day + age 40	5	
Lifestyle sedentary job without exercise	2 – 3	2 – 3
stressful	no conclusive studies	
Family history of premature CAD	high	high
Obesity suggests other risk factors		

Smoking without doubt increases the risk of developing CAD. The patient is more likely to believe the nurse who sets a good example, especially the nurses who have given up smoking themselves. Point out that athletes and most doctors do not smoke, that smoking damages the heart and lungs, and that it is expensive!

Patients with *diabetes* or *hypertension* should be encouraged to maintain control and adhere to medical treatment. It is especially important for these patients to reduce other risk factors, such as obesity and smoking.

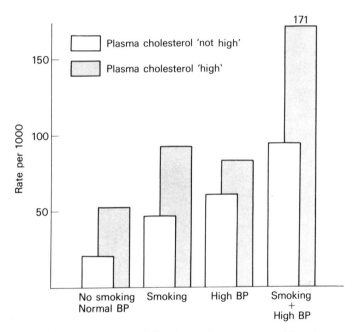

Fig. 7.3 Comparison of the risks of cigarette smoking, hypertension and cholesterol levels in coronary artery disease. Data from the Health Education Council using a ten year study of US males aged 30 – 59.

High *serum lipids* and *cholesterol* levels can be reduced by a diet low in saturated animal fat and high in polyunsaturated vegetable fats. This change in diet is recommended for people who have high serum levels or a family history of premature CAD, as cholesterol intolerance and hyperlipidaemia is familial. Clofibrate may be prescribed for these people. The dietician and nurses should discuss and plan how to change the diet for the better, without increasing food cost or preparation time.

The contraceptive pill has not been shown to be a risk to otherwise healthy women under 40 who do not smoke and who have no family history of CAD.

Obesity has not in itself been proved to be a risk factor, but hypertension, diabetes, and hyperlipidaemia may be precipitated. If an obese person does develop myocardial infarction or other illness, they are more at risk of developing complications of bed rest and will require a longer convalescent period. The dietician and staff should help the patient and his family to a better diet. Alcohol in moderation does not cause coronary artery disease, but it is high in calories.

Stress is not a proven risk factor but increases adrenaline output, which contributes to sugar and fat in the blood and thus to platelet stickiness. Discuss this with the patient and family and try to identify any means by which anxiety and stress can be relieved at work or home. The social worker may also be able to help any specific home or work problems.

A *family history* of cardiovascular disease may be a risk factor, or the risk may be the inherited lifestyle, over-eating, and anxious personality. Patients' families should be encouraged to critically assess their health, diet, exercise, and smoking habits — although in the end the motivation to alter his habits and lifestyle must come from the patient. The patient is more likely to discuss his anxieties with the nurse than with doctors on a formal medical round. Promote discussion between the patients and their families and provide pamphlets and articles (available from the Health Education Council).

Lack of exercise is seen as a risk factor for developing CAD because the unfit body will not be able to make the best use of the oxygen supplies to it — this includes the heart muscle itself. Unfit people have a higher resting heart rate than trained individuals, and their heart rates rise quicker on any exertion; they are therefore more likely to experience angina with even minimal coronary artery stenosis. Angina sufferers can improve their fitness and, though this will not reduce the atheroma or cholesterol levels, their angina will not be precipitated so easily. Three months after myocardial infarction, patients can undertake exercise training and regain the same level of heart work capacity as age-matched sedentary people. Exercise training programmes for people with CAD should begin cautiously under medical direction, with treadmill exercise ECG testing if possible. The type of exercise, its intensity, and frequency should be considered. Walking, jogging, swimming and bicycling all require repetitive and continuous use of the leg muscles. These exercises allow the patient to go at his own pace and are of more cardiovascular benefit than tennis or football for example.

To achieve a training effect on the heart, i.e. lower resting pulse and increase oxygen utilization, exercises should be carried out for at least 20 minutes three times a week. During this time the heart should be maintained at the rate of 220 minus the patient's age, or at a level just lower than that which produced symptoms or ECG changes during exercise testing.

The nursing role in CAD

CAD causes heart failure, ischaemic cardiomyopathy, angina, myocardial infarction, and death in large numbers of the population. There are many old wives' tales about heart disease, and these may cause fear and unnecessary suffering to those who suspect that the pain in their chest is due to coronary heart disease. Reassurance is therefore invaluable. It is worth pointing out that angina does not always lead to myocardial infarction. Following diagnosis and without specific treatment, the mortality is 4% per year but most patients can be controlled on medication or have surgery to live full and active lives.

The nurse must also help the patient to relieve or avoid the pain of angina, and to maintain as full and active a life as possible with or without the use of glyceryl trinitrate (GTN). Education to understand the disease (and so eliminate aggravating or risk factors) is very important for the patient and his family, as is knowledge and confidence about what to do in the event of an attack of angina. Should angina occur, prompt reversal is especially important to prevent arrhythmias and possible tissue damage to the brain, kidneys and myocardium. Relief of the severe pain and anxiety is also mandatory so that the patient does not lose all self-confidence and live in constant fear of another attack and possible death.

PAIN IN CAD

Signs
The following signs may be observed: anxiety — pained expression, lying quietly in bed or a chair, rubbing a hand or clenched fist over his sternum, pale, sweaty, anorexic, nauseous, vomiting, altered respiration — fast or shallow, paralysis of fingers and heaviness of arm which may prevent the patient using the nurse call bell, and rhythm changes noted at the pulse or monitor. Blood pressure may be low with severe pain or raised with the anxiety, and ST segment and T wave changes may be noted on the monitor or 12 lead ECG.

Symptoms
The patient will describe at least one of the following symptoms: *onset* precipitated by exercise, emotion, large meal, cold weather, even at rest;

character of pain as dull heavy ache to an excruciatingly severe constricting pain in centre of chest; *radiation* spreading like a tight, choking, constricting band round the chest, down the left and possibly the right arm to fingers. Pain may spread to or begin in jaw, back, or abdomen; *relieved* by rest, standing or sitting still, and sublingual GTN only; *duration* from 30 seconds to 20 minutes. Over this time suspect myocardial infarction or other cause; *breathlessness* may precede, accompany, or follow pain; and *palpitations* may precede or accompany pain (*see* Fig. 4.1).

Management of CAD

This is directed towards improving the quality of the patient's life and protecting against myocardial infarction. A period of several days' rest at home or in hospital is advisable following the initial onset of angina. Lighter or part time work may be encouraged for a few patients to prevent oxygen demand exceeding supply (*see* p. 176). At the moment there is no proven effective medical therapy that removes or reduces the atheroma already present. Treatment is aimed at reducing the oxygen demands of myocardial muscle, and either preventing or relieving pain to allow the continuation of normal activities.

Beta adrenergic receptor blocking agents block the adrenaline-like responses of the heart to exercise, thereby reducing heart work and lowering oxygen consumption. They act on the sinus node, AV node, and myocardium to reduce heart rate, conduction, contractility and irritability. However, they also produce bronchial constriction and arteriolar vasodilation. Some drugs are more cardiac selective by blocking beta 1 receptors only, so causing less bronchospasm and hypotension (*see* p. 109).

Sudden vasodilation following GTN administration quickly relieves or prevents pain since with a reduction in peripheral resistance, the left ventricle is off-loaded and preload reduced. Sublingual GTN 0.5 mg is absorbed and effective in 1 – 2 minutes, although minor side-effects include flushing, headaches, and possible hypotension and faintness initially. Two or three tablets can be taken at one time. The patient should be reassured that these are not addictive and that in any one day they should take as many tablets as needed. Tablets can be taken prophilactically prior to exercise or other known precursor of the patient's pain. Unfortunately the effect of each tablet does not last for long. Sublingual or oral isosorbide has a slightly stronger and longer-lasting effect. Other long-acting drugs are available, but are not as effective. They may be used in conjunction with GTN.

Nifedipine is a drug that causes vasodilation to peripheral vessels and specifically to the coronary arteries, so it helps angina and prevents coronary spasm. Coronary spasm gives the same symptoms as CAD angina but, on angiography, no narrowing can be seen to explain the pain. An ergometrine test may be performed on these patients. This involves giving a dose of intravenous ergometrine while watching the ECG monitor and the patient. ST segment or T wave changes as well as the characteristic chest pains may occur. GTN and nifedipine should be at hand in case severe coronary artery spasm is induced.

The nurse should assess the patient's general condition including skin colour and warmth, the degree of anxiety, distress, shock and dyspnoea. Observe the heart rhythm by feeling the pulse or by watching the monitor where alterations in rhythm and ST or T wave changes may be noticed. Quietly reassure the patient by staying with him, making him comfortable and relaxed in bed, and giving sublingual GTN or isosorbide as prescribed. If there has been no diagnosis of the chest pain, record a 12 lead ECG.

Notify the doctor immediately if the pain is very severe, if the patient becomes shocked, or if the pain is not relieved by rest and GTN in 15 minutes. For severe pain, intravenous beta blockers and/or diamorphine 5 mg will be given, and possibly oxygen administration may help. The patient should either be closely observed, monitored, or both. If arrhythmias are present, these will be treated with intravenous drugs. Beta blocking drugs may be started or increased and restriction of the patient's mobility with or without sedation may be ordered.

To aid diagnosis and management, attacks of angina should be documented in the nursing records, including the precipitating factors, charater, duration, and relieving factors. Early angiography and possibly coronary artery bypass surgery may be arranged. If the pain continues the IABP (*see* p. 129) may also be considered.

Whether treated by medical or surgical therapy, the patient should be advised how to improve his prognosis by reducing the risk factors and becoming physically fitter.

Surgical treatment

Surgical bypass of the atheromatous plaques is indicated for two groups of patients.
1 Those in whom angina limits their work and life in spite of maximal medical therapy.
2 Those who are shown on angiography to have significant stenosis of the left main coronary or stenosis of three other coronary arteries and whose life expectancy is thus reduced.

Careful noting of the patient's history is essential to identify those who will benefit from surgery, e.g. patients with recent-onset angina which is quickly progressing, or with pain on minimal exertion or even at rest are likely to proceed to myocardial infarction unless surgery intervenes.

Angiography will be carried out, which is itself not without risk but will clearly show the state of the coronary arteries and any narrowings. Best surgical results are obtained from bypassing stenoses through which, at angiography, dye had passed to fill the vessel beyond, or where retrograde filling from a collateral vessel had occurred.

Patients with disease of distal vessels will often be advised against surgery as the results are poor; this will probably include those with diabetes and ischaemic cardiomyopathy. Those patients who are shown to have good left ventricular function at angiography and no other major systemic illness, have a low operative mortality rate, less than 1%. Patients with poor left ventricular function or who have severe diabetes, renal disease or cerebral vascular disease are a higher operative risk.

CAD case study

Mr Richards, a 42-year-old married man with two young children, worked as a car mechanic. He worked hard, smoked 20 – 30 cigarettes a day, and consumed one or two pints of beer a day. He looked fit for his age but was a little overweight since he had given up playing football. He was referred to the cardiological outpatient department by the General Practitioner whom he had visited following several attacks of pain experienced while at work.

His ECG looked normal, he was in regular sinus rhythm rate 90 per minute, blood pressure was 140/90 and a chest X-ray showed clear lung fields with a normal sized heart. When questioned about the pain, Mr Richards was able to answer that this started in the centre of his chest and then spread to his throat, but did not go to his back or down his arms. The pain seemed to come on when he was doing particularly heavy work, but he was not really breathless and did not have palpitations. Whenever he had the pain he would stop what he was doing, and then the pain went in a few minutes. The last few times he had noticed that he had started sweating with the pain and a workmate had said how awful he looked. It was the workmate who had suggested he should go to the doctor. When asked, he also remembered the indigestion-type discomfort he had been having lately, which was not always related to his meals. An exercise ECG was performed which was positive.

Mr Richards was told that his pain and discomfort were due to angina; he was prescribed propranolol 40 mg t.d.s. and glyceryl trinitrate and was instructed how to take these to relieve and avoid pain. He was advised to take a week off work and to report to his General Practitioner if the symptoms did not improve, so that his treatment could be altered. Because of his young age and the recent onset of his angina he was put on the waiting list for angiography.

After returning to work he continued to have some pain and discomfort which he found the GTN relieved almost instantly. He attended outpatients after one month, and in six weeks he was admitted for coronary angiography and a left ventricular angiogram. These revealed that, though his left ventricular function was good, he had over 50% stenosis of the left anterior descending artery, circumflex, and right coronary artery.

Surgery to bypass the stenosed coronary arteries was advised.

MYOCARDIAL INFARCTION

One of the manifestations of coronary artery disease is myocardial infarction (MI), which may or may not have been preceded by recognized angina. The infarction may occur suddenly and unexpectedly and need not be related to any sudden activity or emotion. Infarction can occur at rest, during sleep, and when a lowered blood pressure is insufficient to perfuse diseased coronary arteries, e.g. the hypotension caused by trauma or general anaesthetic.

Infarction (death of tissue) occurs when the demands for oxygen by the myocardium cannot be met. This can be due to complete occlusion of the coronary artery to the muscle by the atheroma process, by thrombi from an atheromatous plaque, or rarely from vegetations from a diseased aortic or mitral valve. A dissecting aortic aneurysm can involve the coronary arteries to give angina or infarction.

Diagnosis

This can be made from the patient's history, the ECG, and from estimation of the cardiac enzymes.

HISTORY

Using the patient's description of the pain, its character and duration, the extreme tiredness, shock or collapse, together with the physical signs can often provide a positive diagnosis before the ECG or cardiac enzymes confirm this. The patient can be told that confirmation of MI takes 2 – 3 days of blood tests and serial ECG s. If positive, the patient will remain in hospital for about 7 – 10 days and convalesce at home for a further 6 – 8 weeks. If the pain is not proven to have been an MI but only an angina attack, the three days' rest will benefit the angina and the patient will be followed-up in the outpatient department after a further few days off work.

The pain of myocardial infarction will be the same as that of angina except that it will last from 20 minutes to several hours. Some patients experience no more than extreme discomfort in their chests, others may have such an excruciating choking pain that they feel they will die. The patient may experience breathlessness or difficulty in breathing, palpitations, extreme anxiety, nausea and even syncope. They will usually look extremely ill and sweat profusely while the pain lasts. The pain will not be relieved by anything except narcotics (*see* Table 4.1).

ECG

The muscle goes through stages of ischaemia and injury before infarction. Following the infarction the muscle become necrosed and over a period of weeks to three months the dead muscle becomes a fibrous scar and does not regenerate. The three stages of ischaemia, injury, and infarction can usually be identified on the ECG. (Right ventricular infarction is uncommon as its oxygen demand and workload are much less than the thick left ventricle.)

Ischaemia and injury of the myocardium affect re-polarization which causes the T waves and ST segments to alter. This can be explained by the current of injury (Fig. 7.4).

Current of injury

The ECG records the flow of electrical current from the heart cells. When resting, the myocardial cells have an equally electrically positive surface charge. No current flows and the ECG shows an isoelectric line. Should a muscle cell be injured that cell will develop a negative surface charge and a current will flow between it and the positively charged healthy cells (Fig. 7.4a).

With myocardial injury, where part of the muscle is injured (sub-endocardial muscle usually remains healthy), a potential difference will exist between the negative surface of the injured cells and the positive surface of the healthy cells. A current will flow. This current in the resting state will cause a depression on the isoelectric line on the ECG trace (Fig. 7.4a). This will, of course, not be noticeable until all the tissues become equally negatively charged (Fig. 7.4b).

When the healthy tissue is electrically stimulated (point 1) depolarizing it until repolarization is complete (point 2) all the myocardial cells will be negatively charged. No current will flow until after repolarization when the healthy cells again become positively charged (Fig. 7.4c). The ECG will show an elevated ST segment from an electrode over the site of injured tissue, and a depressed ST segment over the healthy tissue (Fig. 7.5).

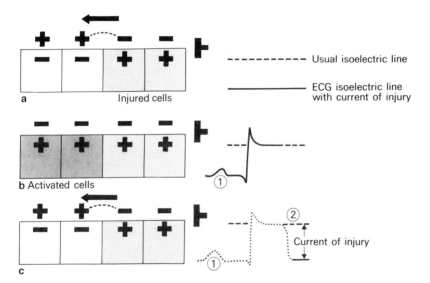

Fig. 7.4   The current of injury (see text for details).

If the myocardium is deprived of blood for six hours or more, tissue death (infarction) will result in permanent Q waves developing on the ECG in those leads over the dead tissue. An area around the infarction will be ischaemic giving typical ST segment and T wave changes (Fig. 7.6). These signs will resolve but the Q wave will remain. The wide Q wave occurs in leads over the infarcted tissue because dead tissue is electrically silent and acts like a window (Fig. 7.7). This means that the electrode will see no impulse vectors coming towards it, only the vectors on the opposite side of the heart going away (Fig. 7.8).

From these signs on the ECG the nurse can localize the infarction and decide if it is recent or old. With this knowledge she will then know what signs and complications to look for (Figs. 7.9 – 7.12).

For the above reasons patients suspected of MI have 12 lead ECG s taken on admission and daily for three days to confirm infarction has occurred and to localize it. To ensure resolution of infarction and ischaemia, ECG s are taken prior to discharge and at outpatient clinic. They are also recorded should the patient experience more pain or any other complication.

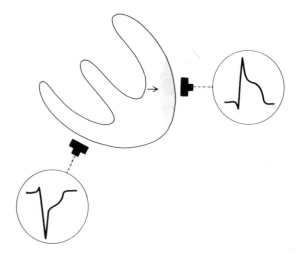

Fig. 7.5   An elevated ST reading over the site of injured tissue and a depressed reading over the healthy tissue.

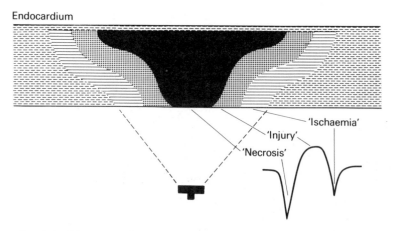

Fig. 7.6   Diagrammatic representation of the Q wave of necrosis, the ST elevation of injury, and the T wave inversion of ischaemia.

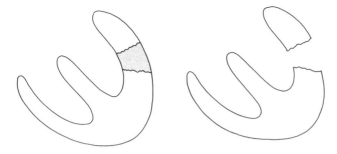

Fig. 7.7   The window effect of a trans-mural infarct.

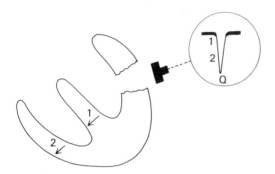

Fig. 7.8   The Q wave resulting from the window effect.

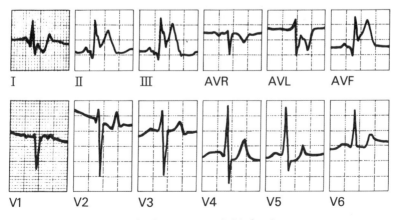

I	II	III	AVR	AVL	AVF
V1	V2	V3	V4	V5	V6

Fig. 7.9   12 lead ECG of inferior myocardial infarction.

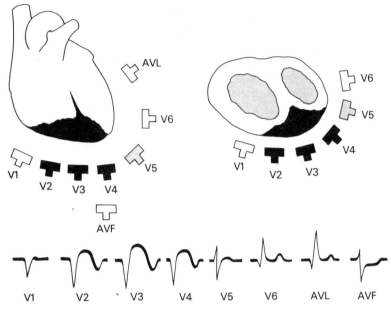

Fig. 7.10   Acute anteroseptal myocardial infarction.

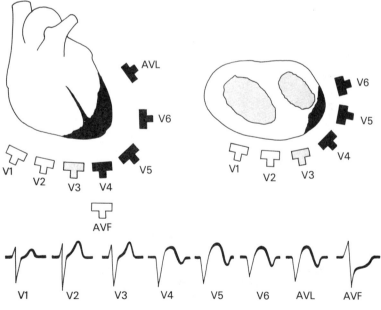

Fig. 7.11   Acute anterolateral myocardial infarction.

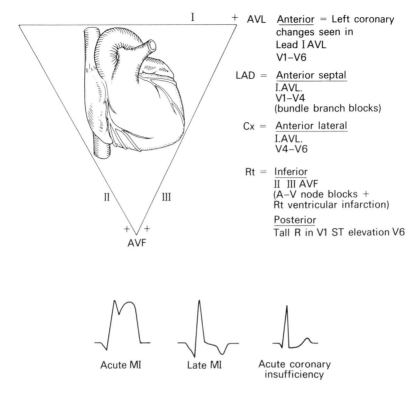

Fig. 7.12 Localization of myocardial infarction from the ECG leads. LAD = left anterior descending, Cx = circumflex.

CARDIAC ENZYMES

To confirm MI has occurred and to indicate its extent and timing, biochemical blood tests for raised serum enzymes are made. The dying muscle releases these enzymes into the bloodstream but, since other dying or injured tissues also release enzymes, tests to indicate specific cardiac muscle death are carried out. The different enzymes are released at different intervals, so the infarction can be dated and any extension of infarction clearly identified.

CPK

Creatinine phosphokinase is also released from brain and skeletal muscle and will therefore be raised following intramuscular injections, surgery, or bruising which might have occurred if the patient had collapsed and fallen. It is the first enzyme to rise after myocardial infarction and is therefore useful to detect infarction quickly in case the patient is being considered for angiography or cardiac surgery. If infarction has occurred, surgery will not usually be carried out immediately. This is because the risks of surgery are higher post infarction than if the patient is conservatively managed for at least six weeks to allow the infarction to settle before operation. CPK is raised after six hours, peaks at 12 – 20 hours, and is normal after 2 – 4 days.

SGOT

Serum glutamic oxaloacetic transaminase levels rise after 9 – 12 hours and remain elevated for 3 – 7 days following myocardial infarction. It is also raised in kidney, brain, and liver damage and occasionally following pulmonary embolism.

LDH

Lactic dehydrogenase and hydroxbutyric dehydrogenase (HBD) rise and peak after 72 hours and can remain elevated for 5 – 14 days post MI. They are also raised with other tissue and red cell damage (if the sample is haemolysed, for example).

Management

The nursing management of MI must respond to a number of potential patient problems.

Heart work will be increased by pain and anxiety because they will provoke catecholamine release to give a tachycardia and vasoconstriction. Physical exertion of any kind will obviously also increase the work demanded of the heart.

Arrhythmias will cause an increase in heart work and can cause heart failure or sudden death.

Mechanical defects of the left ventricle will reduce its efficiency and cause it to fail. Infarction of a large portion of the left ventricular muscle may reduce cardiac output below a level sufficient to adequately perfuse all the tissues. Cardiogenic shock may result (*see* p. 125).

An infarcted septum may rupture to give a septal defect, this will cause pulmonary oedema and low cardiac output.

Infarction of papillary muscle may lead to rupture of a chordae tendineae or papillary muscle. This will cause gross mitral valve regurgitation to also give pulmonary oedema and a low cardiac output.

Infarcted myocardium will necrose, then over six weeks to three months it will fibrose. If a full thickness infarction has occurred, the myocardium may rupture at the necrosis stage, usually resulting in death, or an aneurysm may form at the fibrosis stage.

Thrombi may form in fibrillating atria or poorly contracting ventricles. Platelets will aggregate on the roughened surface over infarcted areas, but a clot is particularly likely to form in an aneurysmal sac. Emboli from the left heart will travel to any organ, the brain, gut, kidneys or limbs, to cause death of tissue with a variety of signs and symptoms that will require urgent attention.

Renal failure may occur if the blood pressure falls below the patient's critical level, about 80 or 90 mmHg systolic, resulting in retention of water, urea and potassium.

The problems associated with *bed rest* must be guarded against — venous thrombosis, pulmonary emboli, pressure necrosis, chest infection, constipation and depression. The loss of independence and confidence can result in the person becoming permanently dependent on others, and convinced that they will always be an invalid.

Treatment

Since CAD is the commonest heart condition that the nurse is likely to encounter, its treatment will be discussed in some detail. This is based on conservative management that relies almost entirely on skilled nursing care. There are five main objectives:

1 Relief of pain and anxiety.
2 Prevention of infarction extension and heart failure.
3 Early detection and treatment of complications and arrhythmias.
4 Prevention of complications of bed rest.
5 Return to a full and active life.

PAIN RELIEF

The pain of myocardial infarction is very often severe, causing catecholamine release, anxiety, and shock. Intravenous diamorphine 5 mg is usually effective and this route is preferred because the pain is relieved immediately, whereas intramuscular drugs may take a long time to be effective because of the low cardiac output with poor tissue perfusion. In addition, if enzyme measurements of CPK are required, i.m. injections can invalidate the results by causing muscle damage. Following myocardial infarction, i.v. diamorphine causes less nausea and respiratory depression than other narcotics. Many doses can be given without the risk of addiction.

The pain dulls to an ache for 2 – 3 days and oral analgesics such as Distalgesic may be effective, but the nurse must consider if the pain indicates further angina threatening an extension of the infarction. After 2 – 3 days the pain may be due to pericarditis caused by infarction to the epicardial surface. A pericardial rub will be heard by stethoscope, the pain will be worse in different positions and on deep inspiration, and will be relieved by leaning forward. Indomethicin or aspirin will relieve the inflammation and pain. This pericarditis may become very severe up to three months, requiring steroids and narcotic analgesics (Dressler's syndrome). The patient will require explanation concerning these pains to reassure him it is not a further 'heart attack' occurring.

PREVENTION OF INFARCTION EXTENSION AND HEART FAILURE

Oxygen supply and demand can be balanced by resting the mind and body. On admission, put the patient quietly to bed in a comfortable position, in his own night clothes. A friendly, unhurried but efficient manner should help to allay anxiety. Explain in simple language any nursing or medical procedures such as monitoring, oxygen administration and an i.v. cannula as routine for all those with chest pain. The patient is usually rested in bed for 24 – 48 hours, but he may stand out of bed to use the bottle or commode. Bed bathing and lifting should be carried out using two nurses for a heavy or ill patient to prevent the patient exerting himself.

Patients may be visited at any time by two or three close members of the family or friends, who are advised to let the patient rest as much as possible and to avoid mention of anxieties about home or work. A social worker may be able to help or advise the family with any money or domestic problems. If the patient is very ill, the spouse may be offered overnight hospital accommodation if any is available.

Catecholamine release in shocked states vasoconstricts bloodflow to the splanchnic areas so that digestion, absorption, and gut motility are reduced. Nausea and vomiting may result. To rest the gut and prevent a large part of the cardiac output being diverted to the gut after a heavy meal, a light diet should be offered. To increase rest and to lower metabolic needs, night sedation is usually offered; many cardiologists also prescribe sedatives such as diazepam throughout the day.

EARLY DETECTION AND TREATMENT OF COMPLICATIONS

Patients suspected of MI are usually admitted to a coronary unit where trained nurses can closely observe them. The patient is immediately connected to a cardiac monitor, so that potentially life-threatening arrhythmias can be identified and promptly treated.

Most patients who suffer a myocardial infarction die from arrhythmias before they reach hospital. Ordinary ambulances carry neither the equipment nor the suitably trained personnel to identify and reverse arrhythmias or cardiac arrest. To meet this need, some hospitals equip special vehicles and make medical personnel available to take a *mobile coronary unit* to the patient, stabilize their condition, then carefully transport them to hospital. In some areas doctors go with the ambulance, in other areas ambulance personnel or nurses are trained to carry out arrhythmia identification, insertion of intravenous lines, administration of drugs according to a protocol, intubation, and defibrillation. Patients who are admitted via casualty with suspected MI should be transferred immediately to a coronary care unit.

Myocardial infarction means death of heart muscle that cannot regenerate. Any increase in the size of the infarction can cause death or increase the convalescence period. An extensive infarction will restrict the patient's lifestyle with recurrent heart failure likely in spite of innumerable drugs. On the other hand, a patient with a small infarction can return to a full life with no medication or restrictions. Any further pain or other symptoms that the patient experiences should therefore be investigated and treated, as outlined below.

A *raised temperature* to about 38.5° C indicates that tissue damage has occurred, but this should resolve in 3 – 4 days. A persistent temperature could indicate pericarditis, infarction extension, deep vein thrombosis, pulmonary embolism, or a chest infection. A raised white cell count would be found in all these conditions.

Heart rate and rhythm should be observed continually for signs of any arrhythmia. The nurse should record the apex beat for a full minute every hour to detect rhythm disturbances. If the patient is not monitored, the heart rhythm can be ascertained by listening to the apex beat or feeling the pulse. If irregularly irregular it is usually atrial fibrillation, if dropped beats occur, ventricular ectopics or second degree heart block can be suspected. An ECG tracing will confirm the rhythm. A patient with a persistent tachyardia should be mobilized more gently until it resolves because it may indicate or precipitate heart failure. Whether or not the patient is symptomatic, the doctor should be notified of any dangerous, or potentially dangerous, arrhythmias, e.g. extreme bradycardias, heart blocks, supraventricular tachycardia, ventricular ectopics, and ventricular tachycardia (*see* pp. 58–80).

An increase in *respiratory rate* indicates heart failure. This could be due to an arrhythmia or left ventricular failure. Alternatively chest infection often occurs in elderly patients with even mild heart failure on bed rest, due to the presence of fluid in the lungs and the lack of movement causing hypostatic bronchial pneumonia.

The *blood pressure* is usually lowered following myocardial infarction, to the extent that those previously on hypotensive drugs may never need them again. However, a pressure below 90 mmHg systolic may not be adequte to perfuse vital organs, especially the myocardium and kidneys. Estimations of blood electrolytes and urea are carried out on admission and at intervals. Patients receiving diuretics are particularly prone to electrolyte imbalance, which can cause myocardial irritation to precipitate ventricular arrhythmias, or cause lethargy with muscle weakness.

The *fluid balance* and urine output must therefore be carefully recorded to detect low kidney perfusion caused by hypovolaemia or low blood pressure. Fluid retention occurs in response to stress and heart failure and can overload the heart and tissues to give pulmonary oedema; fluids are therefore often restricted to 1.5 litres per day initially. More accurate measurements of body and heart fluid requirements using central venous pressure monitoring or a Swan – Ganz pulmonary arterial line can be useful in sick patients (*see* p. 11).

POSSIBLE COMPLICATIONS OF BED REST

As previously detailed (pp. 105 & 113) rest in bed is an important part of the treatment of many heart conditions as it reduces heart work. However, stasis of venous blood, reduction of gut motility, and mental frustration can cause problems and, as soon as the pain and any immediate life-threatening conditions have been dealt with, the nursing staff should institute care to prevent any further insult to the patient's body or senses — including thromboemboli, chest infection, pressure necrosis and digestive upsets.

Despondency about the future and the possible length of time off work can cause depression and increase lethargy. The patient and his family must be kept informed of probable progress and any treatment, and should be encouraged to plan ahead positively but realistically. In the time between rest periods, meals and nursing activities the patient should be encouraged to participate in non-exertional pastimes such as conversation, watching television or playing cards.

Early mobilization should also be encouraged because it has been found that prolonged periods of bed rest following infarction do not improve prognosis. Indeed the thromboemboli and other bed rest complications endanger recovery.

RETURN TO A FULL AND ACTIVE LIFE

Ward mobilization
Rehabilitation begins from the moment of admission. While monitoring,

oxygen, and intravenous infusions are started, the nurse should give the patient some idea of the time he will be on the monitor and bed rest, and encourage him to plan ahead to the next 7 – 10 days of hospitalization prior to discharge.

After 24 hours of no pain or arrhythmias, the patient can sit out in a chair and monitoring can be discontinued. Coronary units with progressive care areas are ideal but, in many hospitals, patients are moved from the coronary unit to a medical ward. Explanation, reassurance, and introduction to the new ward and staff should be full to ensure continuity of care.

Transient heart failure is common for the first few days but, if this is mild, this should not delay non exertional activites, such as walking to the toilet and joining other patients at the meal table.

Persistent tachycardia, third heart sound, and basal crepitations all suggest heart failure. Diuretics may be prescribed. These patients will be allowed to progress more slowly otherwise the increased oxygen demands on the myocardium may not be met, so causing infarction extension.

Recurrence of angina warns of threatening infarction extension. Beta adrenergic blocking agents, such as propranolol, may be prescribed, as well as a slower programme of mobilization. Heavy activities or work are therefore contraindicated until after angiography in case coronary artery bypass surgery is needed to avert another, perhaps fatal, myocardial infarction. If the angina can be controlled by propranolol and GTN, the patient will be discharged and re-admitted after six weeks for angiography. Angiography and surgery can be carried out sooner if absolutely necessary but the mortality and morbidity are much higher than if the heart is given time to recover from the first infarction.

By 7 – 10 days after infarction, most patients will be fully active in the ward; showering or bathing unaided, eating all meals at the table, and walking confidently up and down a flight of stairs without pain or breathlessness. An afternoon rest on the bed should still be encouraged, because the patients are usually woken early and night time disturbances in a ward do occur.

Drugs
On discharge, the patient may have drugs to take including, for example, beta blockers, diuretics, digoxin, anti-arrhythmics, anticoagulants, and glyceryl trinitrate. These should be clearly explained to the patient and spouse, the labels checked, and example times given. Hospitals usually give a 3 – 7 day supply only. It should be stressed which tablets must be continued, and how the patient obtains more. A letter will be sent to the patient's General Practitioner, and the patient and family should be

encouraged to contact their doctor if at all worried. The doctor may then make arrangements for an earlier outpatient appointment or re-admission.

Exercise
The amount of exercise should be clearly outlined, 'Take it easy' is no advice; most patients should plan a return to full activities in 4 – 8 weeks, including work. An outline for activities is given below.

Week 1 Continue as when in hospital, light meals, rest after lunch on the bed, early night. 'No heavy housework' means no cooking or cleaning, but washing-up or making a hot drink would be suitable. Walk in the garden, but no gardening.

Week 2 Depending on the individual's feeling of fitness, and allowing for rests when tired, short walks, but no shopping or use of public transport. Plenty of rest is still needed.

Week 3 More active about the house, walking to nearby shops. Visiting neighbours if desired. Up all day with a shorter afternoon rest in a chair.

Week 4 1 or 2 mile walk, using public transport, light housework, some cooking, light gardening, working at home. An outpatient visit is usually planned for 4 – 6 weeks.

For women especially, a period at a convalescent home is encouraged, unless a member of the family can stay at home to care and morally support the patient for 2 – 3 weeks. Discuss this with the patient and family — a stay with certain relatives may not be restful.

Tiredness is a predominant feature, which the patient should be prepared for. Some patients require help from the social worker or doctor to obtain part time or light work (permanently or temporarily) until they feel fully fit. Many older patients choose early retirement, but should be encouraged to remain as active as possible. Only a few patients require prolonged convalescence and assistance, including help with bathing from the District Nursing Services, and Home Help from Social Services.

After 8 – 12 weeks, if the patient is otherwise fit, an individual exercise training programme could be started (*see* p. 180).

Outpatients
A visit is arranged usually 4 – 6 weeks post discharge. Examination will include a 12 lead ECG to check for resolving ST segment and T wave changes. Persistent ST elevation and a dilated border of the left ventricle on chest X-ray indicate left ventricular aneurysm formation.

Physical examination will include listening for signs of heart failure in the lungs and heart, estimating jugular pressure and looking for signs of peripheral oedema. Discussion is an important part of the visit to reveal progress: whether any pain, breathlessness, palpitations or dizziness occur and to what these symptoms are related. Drugs will be reviewed and many discontinued. If symptoms are occurring, the patient may be further investigated as an in- or an outpatient; angiography, echocardiography, exercise ECG, or 24 hour cassette monitoring with a view to surgery or drug treatment may be carried out.

Patients are usually encouraged to resume work or full activities if they have no heart failure or pain. Some patients, particularly the elderly, need 3 – 9 months before they feel fully well and confident. Those who have had large or repeated infarctions may remain in heart failure and only manage reduced activities.

MI case study

Mrs Johns was a 58-year-old canteen worker in a hospital. One day at lunchtime she was noticed by the Nursing Officer to be rather pale and quiet, not her usual cheerful self. Mrs Johns then admitted that she did have a rather persistent pain in her chest, which she was sure would go when she was able to sit down after lunch.

Mrs Johns was persuaded to sit down there and then. She was relieved because she felt very tired, and a little worried about the pain. It transpired that she had been having these pains for several weeks, but they usually only lasted for 5 or 10 minutes, but this one had been going on for nearly three hours. When asked to describe the pain, she rubbed her fist over the lower half of her sternum and said that the pain was more a heavy constricting feeling than a pain. It started in the centre of her chest, through to her back and down the left arm, even making her fingers feel tingly and the arm weak. The catering officer was informed and Mrs Johns was put in a wheelchair and taken to the coronary unit where a 12 lead ECG revealed typical changes of an inferior myocardial infarction.

Chapter 8
Cardiac surgery

Indications for surgery

Cardiac surgery is carried out to relieve debilitating symptoms or to improve life expectancy. Surgery greatly improves the lives even of patients in their 60s and 70s, allowing them to be healthy and independent. However, these elderly people have a higher risk of developing operative and post-operative complications. The commonest operations are for valvular, congenital, or ischaemic heart disease.

Worsening heart failure, pulmonary symptoms, syncope, episodes of left ventricular failure, or emboli constitute an urgent need for surgery especially in the case of *valve disease*. Some *congenital* defects are inoperable. Palliative methods to increase or decrease pulmonary bloodflow, relieve obstructions, or increase mixing of blood are carried out on infants to protect the lungs and heart from permanent damage and to maintain life. Full corrective procedures are carried out before school age (or when discovered if older) even if the child is asymptomatic. This is to prevent heart failure or pulmonary hypertension and ensure normal growth and development. Surgery is also considered when the patient is unable to lead a normal life because of *angina*, in spite of medical therapy, or when life expectancy is diminished. Patients with disease of three coronary vessels or narrowing of the left main stem coronary artery will be offered operations, even if their symptoms are not severe and can initially be controlled medically. Post infarction ventricular aneuryms can be exised to treat heart failure, thromboemboli or arrhythmias.

Preoperative investigations

The patient is usually admitted three or four days prior to surgery to allow him to settle into the ward, to allow him and his family to establish a trusting relationship with the staff, and for various tests to be carried out to ensure that he is in an optimal physical and emotional condition for surgery.

The patient's *medical history* will be taken in detail: noting severity, frequency, precipitating, and relieving factors of pain, dyspnoea, fatigue, palpitations, and dizziness. Lung disease may be present, with previous or present asthma, tuberculosis, emphysema or bronchitis. Other diseases that are likely to complicate surgery may be evident, such as hypertension, bleeding or clotting disorders, adrenal insufficiency, recent operations, or infections of other systems. The presence of diabetes, renal or severe lung disease may seriously affect recovery.

The patient may be receiving *drugs*. Digoxin is usually stopped 48 hours prior to operation because toxicity may develop to cause serious arrhythmias, though beta blocking agents are usually continued until operations. Other cardiac or hypotensive drugs will be clearly noted.

The physical examination will reveal the patient's general state of health. The colour of the skin, nail beds, and mucous membranes should be recorded, as well as the pulse rate and volume (note if these are irregular or if an apex pulse deficit exists). Assess the patient's state of hydration and look for oedema. Any sites of infection should be cleared before the operation, and a dental opinion sought, to avoid endocarditis from *Streptococcus viridans*.

The heart will have been investigated prior to surgical referral and the results of angiography, cardiac catheterization, echocardiography and a recent ECG will be reviewed.

Chest X-ray will indicate the heart size and presence of any aneurysms or calcified valves. Raised pulmonary arterial and venous pressure will be shown by increased vascularity of the lungs. Pulmonary effusions, emboli, or infections will be apparent.

Pulmonary function tests may be carried out to identify any restrictive respiratory disorders that could complicate postoperative recovery. It is useful for the anaesthetist to know the patient's normal blood gas level in case the patient develops ventilation problems immediately after the operation. Adults are usually ventilated postoperatively for 6 – 12 hours. If the lungs are known to be abnormal, the anaesthetist and physiotherapist will alter their expectations and treatment accordingly.

Renal function will be tested by measurement of serum urea and electrolytes and a 24 hour urine sample for creatine clearance. Abnormal sodium, calcium and particularly potassium could cause serious cardiac arrhythmias postsurgery. A MSU will be tested for the presence of infection, albumen, casts, and red blood cells as well as routine ward urine testing.

Liver function may be impaired due to prolonged congestion from heart failure. Clotting studies and measurement of prothrombin time will be carried out, and patients on anticoagulant therapy will be very carefully assessed; the drugs will be stopped prior to surgery. Vitamin K may be given to increase prothrobin times two days preoperatively.

Platelet and haemoglobin levels will be measured, and the blood bank notified to cross-match ten units of blood. Other blood tests of glucose, Australia antigen and Wasserman reaction are taken. The patient's height and weight are used to calculate the dosage of anaesthetic and cardiac drugs.

Preoperative preparation

If time allows, fluid retention or heart failure will be controlled prior to surgery with diuretics, fluid restriction, and bed rest. It is not usually necessary to give an enema or suppositories before cardiac surgery, but Dorbanex two nights before surgery may be prescribed. A visit from the dietician will be beneficial if the patient has special dietary requirements.

PHYSIOTHERAPY

Chest infection is a real risk following cardiac surgery. The chest will have been opened by a sternal split and the ribs stretched apart. The patient will have been ventilated overnight and have spent the operation time and much of the immediate recovery, lying in one position. Pain and fear of moving or coughing are the main problems. A visit by the physiotherapist prior to surgery allows the patient to practice deep breathing and coughing exercises, and to build a trusting relationship with the physiotherapist. If inhalation therapy using a Bird or Bennett respirator or steam inhalations are to be used, the patient is shown how to use these.

EMOTIONAL PREPARATION

Cardiac surgery is commonly reported in the media and many people have a distorted perception or fear of what is involved. The nurse, medical, and paramedical staff must therefore work as a team to prepare the patient emotionally as well as physically. The patient and the family should be given an honest and straightforward appraisal of the benefits and risks of the operation.

Some patients have been suffering from symptoms for many months or years, and look forward to the relief offered by operation. These patients and their families will also have had time to come to terms with the fact of having heart disease, and may look upon the operation and the possible risks philosophically and calmly.

Other patients who have had a more acute illness may be very anxious, irritable and withdrawn, making it more difficult to prepare them emotionally. These patients may feel lonely and isolated in an alien hospital world, but it is most important that their cooperation and trust are obtained. The nurse must try to be understanding and supporting, allowing them to explore their feelings without threat of rebuke or ridicule. Some may insist that they want a period of time at home to adjust mentally to the prospect of such a serious operation, even against strong medical advice that an urgent operation is necessary. All the nurse's tact and persuasive power may be needed, but the patients' wishes must be respected and their fears taken seriously. Placing this type of patient in the company of others who have had an uneventful postoperative recovery and who are coping cheerfully and well is an obvious advantage to the patient's mental well-being.

A minister of religion may be able to assist in the spiritual and emotional preparation, and a social worker should be available to help with family arrangements and monetary problems. Arrangements for the period after discharge should be discussed and planned; this may also help the patient to look ahead hopefully.

A doctor will explain the planned operation before the patient signs a consent form, and a senior nurse should explain further and give information to the patient and family concerning the postoperative recovery period, physiotherapy, diet, fluid restriction, visiting, and convalescence. Patient education can be helped with the use of diagrams, booklets, and discussion.

Prior to the operation a nurse from the intensive care unit (ICU) should visit the patient, and parents of children, to discuss the immediate postoperative care. The patient thus has a further opportunity to ask questions and can make requests for the use of dentures, glasses, hearing aid or preferred first name while in the ICU. The nurse can observe the patient's general condition and note any hearing or speech defects. A visit to look at the unit may help some patients.

The patient will probably be ventilated for 6 – 12 hours, and during this time will be unable to speak. Assurance should be given that, while in the ICU, the patient will be assigned a nurse who will be with him at all times; this nurse will know, without the patient speaking, when to give more intravenous sedatives and pain killers, although much of the time the patient will be asleep.

THEATRE PREPARATION

Patients undergoing cardiac surgery not only have their chests opened, but many monitoring devices, drips, and drains are inserted, and major arteries and veins are cannulated to connect the patient to cardiopulmonary bypass. If the femoral artery is used for cannulation, the groin will need shaving and cleansing as well as the chest, axilla, and arms. The operation for coronary artery disease requires the removal of the saphenous vein from one or both legs to bypass the narrowed coronary arteries. Both legs will therefore need shaving and if available, a hospital barber will carry this out. Being careful not to break the skin is important as this lessens the risk of infection.

The patient then bathes and washes his hair using a bactericidal soap. The bath may be repeated on two or three occasions; each time the patient dresses in clean night clothes and returns to clean bed clothes.

The night before surgery the patient will be prescribed *night sedation* to encourage a good night's rest. Nothing to eat or drink will be allowed from six hours before surgery.

On the day of the operation the hospital theatre procedure should be followed meticulously. The patient is thus brought to the theatre by a ward nurse, having been fasted, shaved, washed and relaxed — after an intramuscular injection of a narcotic (e.g. papaveretum) an hour earlier.

OPEN CARDIAC SURGERY

Surgery to the heart itself does not usually take very long. It is the anaesthetic preparation, with insertion of monitoring devices and the linking to and weaning from the cardiopulmonary bypass pump, that make up most of the 3 – 5 hours the patient is in theatre. The theatre team is made of experienced nurses, surgeons, anaesthetists, perfusion and monitoring technicians, and operating department assistants.

The surgeon is unable to operate on a beating heart, so the heart must be stopped and emptied of blood for most procedures. The lungs are allowed to collapse since otherwise they would be in the way of the surgical field. Tissue perfusion and oxygenation are maintained by taking the blood from the venae cavae, passing it through an oxygenator and pumping it back into the aorta.

ECG monitoring, anaesthesia, and artificial ventilation are established in the anaesthetic room; also a radial arterial line to monitor arterial blood pressure, three central venous lines, usually inserted into the external jugular vein, to monitor the central venous pressure and to give fluids and drugs, a naso-pharyngeal temperature probe to record core body temperature, a large-bore peripheral venous line to allow rapid administration of blood and plasma, and a urinary catheter to record urine flow.

The patient is wheeled into theatre, where an extensive iodine skin preparation is carried out and he is draped in sterile towels.

If the procedure is for coronary artery vein bypass grafts, a team of surgeons will carefully remove a section of the saphenous vein from the leg, while another team opens the chest by splitting the whole of the sternum using an oscillating saw that is powered by compressed air. The surgeon will diathermy and tie off bleeding points, then insert a retractor to hold the sternal edges well apart to give a clear view of the heart and lungs. The pericardium is now opened and the heart can be inspected.

Meanwhile, the anaesthetist monitors the patient's vital functions and collects a litre of the patient's own blood into donor transfusion bags, which are allowed to fill by gravity from a central venous line. The blood volume is replaced by a plasma substitute. This removal of blood serves two main purposes. Firstly, when the haematocrit is reduced from 45% to 25%, the circulating blood volume is less viscous, so that when the patient is attached to the cardiopulmonary bypass pump, the blood thus flows more freely causing less destruction to the red cells and platelets as they pass along the tubing. Rouleaux formation is thereby decreased and capillary bloodflow is increased — so reducing the incidence of renal damage. The second function is that the blood removed may be transfused back to the patient at the end of the operation, when all surgical leaks are closed. It is still fresh and contains the clotting factors and platelets that are lacking in blood from the banks.

Cardiopulmonary bypass

The patient is heparinized with 9000 units of heparin per square metre of body surface, which has been calculated from the height and bodyweight. The reservoir of the bypass machine contains two litres of cooled fluid, a mixture of isotonic electrolyte solution and a plasma substitute, e.g. one litre of Hartmann's solution and one litre of Haemocel. This solution further haemodilutes the patient to haemglobin between 7 and 10 g/dl.

The venae cavae are cannulated via the right atrial appendage, the blood flows to the oxygenator where an air and oxygen mixture bubbles through it. The blood is then de-bubbled and cooled before it is pumped to the aorta under a constant pressure and flow control. The aortic cannula is placed above an aortic cross-clamp so that if the coronary arteries are to be perfused, they have separate arterial cannulae from the pump.

Some blood enters the left heart from the bronchial veins so a vent is placed in the left ventricle to entirely empty it. Irreversible damage could occur if the still heart were allowed to distend with blood.

Since the patient has received a large dose of heparin, any blood spilt in the operating field will not clot. This blood can be suctioned clear of the site, filtered and passed into the resevoir of the bypass machine and back to the patient.

The patient is cooled to about 30°C to slow cell metabolism and thus reduce the tissue oxygen requirements during bypass; for this a heat exchanger is incorporated into the bypass machine. The blood will be re-warmed towards the end of the surgery. The perfusion technician will take repeated blood samples for blood gas and pH estimations as well as controlling the flow and pressure of blood to the aorta.

The heart is stopped by emptying it of blood then electrically fibrillating it; alternatively it is cooled and stopped by perfusing the coronary arteries with about 600 ml of *cardioplege*. This is usually ice-cold Hartmann's solution that contains magnesium and a high dose of potassium to 'poison' the heart into asystole. Repeated doses will be given to keep the heart in asystole and at about 4 – 10°C. If cardioplege is used, the coronary arteries do not need intra-operative perfusion with blood.

When the surgeon finishes operating on the heart, the patient is slowly re-warmed. Less blood is taken up from the venae cavae to allow the heart to fill, and the lungs are gently inflated so as not to get in the surgeon's way. If the heart has been opened (e.g. for valve replacement), it is now carefully emptied of all air to avoid air embolism. Decannulation of cardiopulmonary bypass takes place over several minutes, to allow the heart to take over from the pump.

Protamine sulphate is administered to reverse the heparin that was given prior to cardiopulmonary bypass. The heart usually begins to beat as it is re-warmed or a coarse fibrillation responds to defibrillation. The performance of the heart is watched directly in the chest and also on the monitor screen where the ECG, arterial, and venous pressures are displayed. A cannula is inserted into the left atrium and through the chest wall to measure left atrial pressure. This is the filling pressure of the left ventricle so blood is given to maintain this pressure at an adequate level to keep the ventricle optimally primed, but without overfilling the left atrium and causing back pressure to the pulmonary veins and right heart. Inotropic support or pacing may be necessary at this time; the latter will involve inserting transthoracic pacing waves to the atrium and ventricle.

Two drains are placed through separate stab wounds, one to lie retrosternally and the other in the right chest to keep the heart and pericardium free of blood. The drains are attached to underwater seal drainage bottles. The sternum is closed with wire sutures, the subcutaneous tissue with catgut, and the skin with subcuticular sutures of Dexon.

The patient usually remains ventilated for transfer to the intensive care bed. This is a critical period because most of the monitoring devices are temporarily disconnected. The anaesthetist and intensive care nurse recheck measurements of vital functions before the patient leaves the theatre area.

IMMEDIATE POSTOPERATIVE CARE

While the patient is in theatre, in the intensive care unit the postoperative bed and bedsite are prepared against a check list for it is important that they are received into a clean and safe environment. All equipment should be tested to make sure it is in good working order and that connections fit securely. The nurse assigned to the patient's care should:
1 Be knowledgeable as to the safe working of all equipment used.
2 Be able to observe and accurately chart the various parameters measured.
3 Know what changes to look for and how to take appropriate action.
4 Be confident in instituting emergency procedures.
5 Show an awareness of the patient's need for comfort, pain relief and constant reassurance especially if they are ventilated.
6 Be gentle, yet thorough, in carring out basic nursing procedures.
The nurse should be experienced and qualified or a suitably supervised student nurse. Help should always be readily available from a senior qualified nurse and from experienced surgical and anaesthetic staff.

The patient is received from theatre directly onto a bed which has been prepared with a sheepskin, single pillow and the various apparatus to maintain ICU conditions during transport.The patient will initially be covered by a heat-retaining blanket.

Before leaving the theatre area, the nurse should obtain clear instructions from the surgical and anaesthetic staff both about the operation performed and a number of other factors affecting management: intra-operative complications (e.g. arrhythmias or excessive bleeding), the dose and rate of any inotropic support infusions, the presence of any pacing wires, and to what level the venous and arterial presures must be maintained with either blood transfusions or inotropic support.

The patient is attached to a portable monitor and blood pressure gauge. His ventilation is supervised by an anaesthetist, who may hand ventilate the patient with oxygen, or attach him to a miniventilator that is driven by an entonox cylinder. The air entry, chest movement, and endotracheal tube are checked; the heart rhythm and blood pressure are ascertained to be normal. The patient is then quickly and smoothly transferred to the Intensive Care Unit accompanied by a nurse, an anaesthetist and cardiac surgeon. If the journey involves the use of lifts or long corridors, then provision for cardiac or respiratory emergencies must be made. A defibrillator, an oxygen mask, oxygen and bag for hand ventilation should be on the bed.

On return to the ICU, a nurse and an assistant will connect the patient to the prepared monitoring and measuring devices, to intravenous lines, and to the ventilator or oxygen mask. Baseline observations and recordings should be charted (Table 8.1) and the patient settled in 10 minutes.Apart from the surgical aspect of blood loss and replacement, care is directed towards improving cardiac output while maintaining other bodily functions of the lungs, kidneys and brain.

Following surgery, the heart can be considered as being in a state of cardiogenic shock, from which it should recover in 2 – 6 hours. For this reason, frequent observations of parameters that indicate cardiac output and tissue perfusion will be recorded ¼ hourly for two hours, ½ hourly for two hours, then hourly if the patient's condition is satisfactory. These are discussed below.

Table 8.1   Immediate postoperative care of the cardiac patient.

Function	Action
Heart rate and rhythm	Connect to ECG montior
Blood pressure	Connect to transducer and sphygmomanometer
Central venous pressure	Connect to manometer
Mediasternal drainage	Connect to drainage bottles — unclamp + milk catheter
Urine output	Connect to urine bag
Temperatures Peripheral & central	Insert lubricated rectal probe Apply skin probe to foot or big toe
Ventilation	Anaesthetist connects and sets rate, volume and 0_2 %. Checks air entry
Conscious level	Observe pupils. Ask patient to move limbs on command. Reassure and inform patient

HEART RATE

An apex rate of 90 – 120 is usually necessary to maintain a cardiac output after surgery. A rate of 70 may be considered too slow, so the patient will be temporarily paced, using the transthoracic wires inserted during surgery. A persistent tachycardia could be a sign of tamponade, hypovolaemia, heart failure, pain or anxiety.

Ectopic beats may precipitate tachycardias or fibrillation and indicate hypokalaemia, hypoxia, or acidosis. They should be reported along with any other changes in vital signs and treated appropriately.

BLOOD PRESSURE

This is measured from an arterial line in a radial artery that is transduced through thin manometer tubing to a monitor and kept patent with heparinized saline. A conventional cuff and sphygmomanometer may be used in conjunction with this. Blood pressure depends on the cardiac output, peripheral resistance, volume and viscosity of the blood. A pressure of 100 – 120 mmHg systolic is actively aimed at.

Hypotension may cause renal, myocardial, or cerebral ischaemia and could be due to hypovolaemia, hypoxia, acidosis, low serum calcium, tamponade, heart failure or arrhythmias. Other parameters of CVP, temperatures, heart rate, drainage and ventilator function should be checked, which will usually indicate the cause. Appropriate action can then be taken:

CVP low, give blood
Heart rate slow, pace patient
Heart rate fast, overpace or give drugs
Heart failure, infuse inotropic drugs and calcium
For tamponade, unblock drains and possibly open the chest
Ventilator failure, hand ventilate on 100% oxygen, check the tube for kinking in the mouth, and pass a suction catheter down the tube to ascertain patency.

Hypertension may strain suture lines to cause excessive bleeding and should be carefully controlled. Common causes are anxiety and pain; these can be allayed with explanation and intravenous diamorphine 5 – 10 mg, in many doses if necessary. Drugs to vasodilate the arterioles and so lower the blood pressure (and venous pressure) are phentolomine 5 – 10 mg and hydrallazine 10 – 20 mg. If blood pressure control is critical, an infusion of nitroprusside may be given via an infusion pump.

VENOUS PRESSURES AND BLOOD REPLACEMENT

Central venous pressure is measured via an intravenous jugular or subclavian cannula previously inserted in theatre and attached to a fluid manometer which is kept patent with a slow infusion of 5% dextrose or attached to a pressure transducer similar to an arterial line. The surgeon will ask for the CVP to be maintained with blood or plasma to a level that was found to be ideal in theatre, about 8 – 15cmH$_2$0. Remember that if the patient is not ventilated, the pressure in the central vein will be 3 – 5 cm H$_2$O lower than when the patient was ventilated.

A low CVP indicates hypovolaemia due to haemorrhage or vasodilation and blood should be transfused. In an adult, 100 ml of blood can be given rapidly, then the CVP re-checked before giving more. Although blood will be given initially, the haemocrit will indicate when plasma or a substitute should be used instead.

A high CVP indicates volume overload, heart failure, or tamponade. Make sure the CVP line is patent and running freely, then report the high CVP and other changes to the doctor. Diuretics, inotropic support or urgent re-operation may be needed.

Where the CVP does not accurately reflect the filling pressure of the left heart, *left atrial (LA) pressure* monitoring will be carried out in the theatre and may be continued for 12 – 24 hours post surgery, e.g. in sick patients with pulmonary hypertension or right heart failure. The nurse transfuses the patient to the LA presure and not the CVP. The LA line is sewn in position and should be treated with great care. Any air or thrombus entering into the left atrium will cause systemic emboli to the brain or other organs. The line is usually transduced via a low volume continuous flushing device similar to arterial lines. Its wave form plus diastolic, systolic, and mean values can be displayed on a screen. When the line is no longer required it is removed slowly, with a three way tap turned off to the patient to prevent air embolism. After removal, bleeding of up to 200ml from the atrium to the mediastinum commonly occurs, so the mediastinal drains are left in situ until about two hours after the left atrial line has been removed.

URINE OUTPUT

This will be measured hourly via a catheter, even in children, as an adequate output is an excellent indicator that cardiac output is satisfactory. Oliguria or anuria are more often due to a fall in cardiac output and hypotension than to underhydration. If the CVP is low, fluid should be transfused to increase blood pressure and renal perfusion. If the

CVP is normal or high, heart failure or tamponade may be present and diuretics or inotropic support may be given.

Oliguria may also be caused by haemolysis of red cells from the cardiopulmonary bypass machine, septicaemia, or disseminated intravascular coagulation. Prior to oliguria, the urine would probably be dark and contain red cells. This discolouration or an output of less than 30 ml an hour should be immediately reported to the doctor, who may prescribe mannitol or other diuretics.

A large urine output may be due to previous overload, diuretics, or the diuretic phase of recovering renal failure. The nurse must maintain the fluid balance and the CVP with an appropriate fluid. Potassium is lost in the urine so that, if the output is large, frequent supplements will have to be given intravenously to maintain a plasma level of 4 – 5.5 mmol/litre. The doctor will take frequent blood samples for levels and, if renal impairment is suspected, a sample of urine will also be measured for electrolytes. A low serum potassium causes ventricular arrhythmias. The urine catherer is usually removed after 12 – 18 hours.

TEMPERATURE

Toe and rectal probes are attached to an electrical thermometer. As the general condition and cardiac output improves, so will the peripheral temperature. Patients returning from theatre are initially cool, with peripheral and central temperatures of about 30°C. The central temperature usually climbs quickly to 37 – 38°C, the peripheral temperature slowly increases over 4 – 6 hours until it is 35°C. At this point the patient can be considered cardiovascularly quite stable; the heat-retaining blanket can be removed and, if all else is normal, the patient can be turned and washed for the first time post operation.

A falling peripheral temperature clearly indicates vasoconstriction and a fall in cardiac output due to hypovolaemia, heart failure, or tamponade. The peripheral temperature will fall before the blood pressure in impending shock.

CONSCIOUS LEVEL

The patient should be conscious within an hour of returning from theatre. The nurse should speak directly to him, call his name and ask him to move his fingers then toes to each side. If this is possible, it indicates both that the patient is fully alert and cooperative, and that no major cerebrovascular accident (CVA) has occurred intraoperatively. A CVA is more likely in patients who have had valve replacement for calcified valves, or valves with clot and vegetation on them. Clot within a fibrillating atria or poorly contracting ventricle may also embolize. Air emboli after open heart surgery can occur if all air is not meticulously evacuated from the heart prior to closure. If the patient fails to wake, or appears to have one sided muscle weakness, report this to the surgical team. Dexamethazone may be given to reduce any cerebral oedema, and the patient will be more cautiously weaned from the ventilator. Early intervention by the physiotherapist will be required.

DRAINAGE

Two drains are inserted into the mediastinum to collect blood from the pericardium. The drains are attached to underwater seal bottles and to a low pressure suction apparatus. They must be kept patent and free from clot, otherwise blood will collect in the pericardium and prevent the heart from filling adequately. This will cause *cardiac tamponade*, which can occur slowly over a period of a few hours or acutely. An acute tamponade demands that the chest is opened immediately to remove the clots around the atrium.

To keep the drains patent, they are thoroughly milked every 15 minutes with a pair of rollers, or milkers. The drain should be held firmly near its insertion site with one hand and vigorously milked with the milkers in the other hand. The drainage is recorded at least hourly depending on unit policy. An initial blood loss for the first hour may be up to 600ml but this amount should be quickly reduced to 50ml or less per hour by the third hour. The bleeding usually changes to haemoserous fluid after 6 – 12 hours and the drains can be removed after about 12 hours if there is minimal loss of 5 – 10 ml per hour. If the drains suddenly stop draining in the first few hours, it is likely that they are blocked. Vigorous milking or increased suction applied directly may unclot a drain. The surgeon must be notified if it is suspected that a drain is blocked.

EXCESSIVE BLEEDING

This may be due to hypertension, incomplete reversal of the heparin used during bypass, lack of platelets or other clotting factors in the patient's blood, or a dislodged suture or tear in the operative field. Other signs of haemorrhage are tachycardia, restlessness, low CVP, cool peripheries, or low urine output. A chest X-ray may show a mediastinal collection.

Treatment
A blood pressure over 120 mmHg systolic is too high if the patient is bleeding; it should be lowered (*see* p. 209).

Protamine sulphate may be given over 5 – 10 minutes to reverse any remaining heparin.

Platelets and other clotting factors may have been lost with the haemorrhage, and stored blood given by transfusion does not contain many clotting factors. A lengthy operation with a prolonged period of cardio-pulmonary bypass will have damaged platelets, fibrin and red cells.

A transfusion of fresh frozen plasma contains many clotting factors, including prothrombin, that may be deficient due to liver disease. Cyclokapron prevents fibrinolysis, a process that rapidly breaks down formed clot: 0.5 g may be given i.v. to release fibrin for wound clotting. Calcium is necessary for clotting as well as for muscle contraction but is depleted by transfusion of citrated stored blood. It is therefore routinely given after every 3 units of blood transfused.

Fresh blood or platelet concentrate may need to be given if the above measures fail. If all these methods do not stop loss of significant amounts of blood, then the patient will be returned to theatre and the operative field explored.

Sudden massive haemorrhage rarely occurs. If several hundred ml of blood drains over 10 – 15 minutes, the chest should be opened immediately in the unit to stop the bleeding point. Repair to the aorta or coronary vessel can then be carried out. A theatre pack should always be available in the unit for this emergency.

BLOOD AND FLUID BALANCE

Blood, plasma, and plasma derivatives — the colloids — are added together and balanced hourly against blood loss. An adult will accrue a positive colloid balance of a maximum of 1500 – 2000 ml when colloids are given to maintain preset venous pressures. Blood should be accurately measured using a weight scale. Stored blood should be filtered and then warmed before being transfused into a peripheral vein.

The nurse should be alert to the possibility of a transfusion reaction, of rashes, or occasionally the dramatic vasodilation and pulmonary oedema of anaphylactic shock. If this is suspected, all blood and plasma should be stopped, the giving sets changed and the patient given a plasma substitute until the transfusion officer has re-checked the blood and old blood bags against the patient's own blood.

Crystalloid balance
Dextrose 5% is the crystalloid fluid most commonly used since saline can produce pulmonary oedema and water retention. The patient will not usually be taking oral fluids for 12 – 24 hours, so his water intake should be

given intravenously and balanced hourly against urine output and gastric aspiration. An insensible loss of up to 600 ml a day due to perspiration, and to oral and tracheal aspiration should be taken into account by the prescribing doctor. Remember too that the patient will usually have a negative crystalloid balance on the first postoperative day.

Overhydration can lead to cardiac failure and pulmonary oedema and would cause a high CVP reading. Underhydration would lead to vasoconstriction, renal failure, hypotension and tachycardia. Bronchial secretions will thicken and be difficult to aspirate or expectorate. Sputum retention and basal collapse may occur.

VENTILATION

Adults and sick children are usually ventilated for 6 – 12 hours post operatively. The nurse should record the ventilator and humidifier function hourly, and check the patient's colour and chest movement. Endotracheal suction and manual hyperventilation using a Waters' or Ambu bag will be carried out after the first hour, then at intervals according to unit policy, to prevent atelectasis and sputum retention.

Extubation will be considered when the patient is cardiovascularly stable, fully conscious and alert, and not bleeding. Blood gases will be checked to ensure that the oxygen, carbon dioxide and acid – base deficit are within normal limits. The anaesthetist will listen to the patient's chest and examine any postoperative X-ray. The patient will then be suctioned orally and endotracheally, sat upright and attached to a Waters' bag or humidified oxygen supply. The rate and depth of respiration will be observed initially by the anaesthetist, who will probably have to remind the patient to breathe. The nurse then records ¼ hourly observations of tidal volume, respiratory rate, heart rate and blood pressure, while observing the patient's colour, chest movement, and conscious level. Signs of inadequate respiration with rising carbon dioxide include tachycardia, hypertension, pink warm skin, and beads of sweat on the forehead and hands. Hypoxia will cause a rise in heart rate, ectopics, hypotension, and heart failure. If these occur the patient should be hand ventilated and re-attached to the ventilator immediately. If the patient remains well, he will be extubated and given oxygen via a face mask and/or nasal cannulae. The ¼ hourly observations should be continued for two hours or until the patient is quite stable.

ANALGESIA AND SEDATION

These will be necessary, sometimes in large quantities. If the patient is to remain ventilated for several hours, intravenous diamorphine or papaveretum should be given whenever it is needed. Patients frequently require four or more doses within the first two hours.

The nurse should continually reassure the awake patient, keep him orientated by telling him he has had his operation, and is now in the intensive care unit, and what the day and time is. Mention that relatives, if they have phoned, have been told that he is progressing well.

If the patient is not ventilated immediately post operatively, he will still require analgesia and sedation. If the patient is in pain and anxious he will not breathe or cough sufficiently well and may be hypertensive and tachycardic. Small doses of intravenous diamorphine or papaveretum in 1 mg increments can be given, followed by a large intramuscular dose. If the respirations are very depressed by the analgesia and repeated reminders by the nurse to breathe deeply are ineffective, the analgesia can easily be reversed with naloxone.

GENERAL NURSING CARE

Vasoconstriction and low cardiac output states cause a marked reduction in skin perfusion. Patients who have an uneventful operation and a quick postoperative recovery will have been lying on their backs for up to ten hours before they are fit to be turned. Patients who are haemorrhaging or have other complications may not be turned for many more hours. Pressure necrosis is therefore a real problem.

The patient is received from theatre straight onto a sheepskin, and the heels should also be on a sheepskin or elevated and resting on water bags. All patient care, including care of mouth, eyes, urine catheter, skin, and limb movements, must be thoroughly but gently given. When the patient's condition is stable and the blood loss is minimal, he can be safely washed and turned. This should be about six hours postoperatively.

POSTOPERATIVE PROGRESS

The morning after surgery the patient should be fully awake and alert, and his cardiovascular system should have recovered from the insult of surgery. If this is so, blood loss is minimal and the patient is able to breathe well unaided; all lines, drains and tubes will be removed during that first morning, except for an intravenous line which will remain in one day more.

The nurse should constantly reassure, encourage, and inform the patient who can be moved from the ICU to a ward area where close observation is possible. Heart rate, blood pressure, and respiration will be checked hourly for 6 – 12 hours; temperature will be recorded four hourly. If there are no problems, all recordings can be reduced to every two, then four, hours for the next four days, then b.d. until discharge.

There are several potential complications in the postoperative patient, the prevention of which is summarized in Table 8.2 and discussed in greater detail below.

ANALGESIA

Relief of pain is of paramount importance throughout the hospital recovery. For 12 – 18 hours after the operation, narcotic analgesia is used. After this, less potent drugs (such as dihydrocodeine 30 – 60 mg) are used and should be given regularly every four hours orally or intramuscularly. Entonox is an excellent short-acting analgesic and can be used during the removal of intercostal drains. The patient should be given analgesia whether he thinks he requires it or not for the first few days since pain will not only prevent resting, but deep breathing and coughing will be inhibited, so leading to sputum retention and chest infection. Pain will also inhibit the patient from moving about, his limbs will become stiff and more painful to move, he will remain lying or sitting in one position and so develop pressure sores and venous stasis. Venous stasis in the legs and abdomen may lead to venous thrombosis and pulmonary emboli.

If pain is severe, and the patient cannot settle with dihydrocodeine, inform the doctor who will listen for a pericardial friction rub and look for signs of infection that could be causing the pain. Some patients will need extra reassurance that a little pain may be expected when they move or cough, and this does not mean that anything is amiss. Rib pain can be expected for several weeks, but mild analgesia should relieve it. After three days, the patient may only require a milder analgesia of Distalgesic or paracetamol.

The nurse must always be suspicious in case the pain is angina, mediastinal infection, pulmonary embolus, or chest infection. Pericarditis postcardiotomy can occur as an auto-immune reaction, similar to postmyocardial infarction, called Dressler's syndrome. It may develop up to three months after surgery. Anti-inflammatory drugs such as indomethacin or aspirin may relieve the pain, but stronger analgesia and steroids may be required.

RESPIRATORY CARE

Cardiac surgery with its attendant procedures is usually lengthy, the lungs may have been collapsed and not ventilated during cardiopulmonary bypass, and large quantities of blood will have been given. In addition patients who have had cardiac surgery are ventilated and nursed on their backs for several hours. All these factors can lead to poor lung function, sputum retention, atelectasis and pneumonia which are a real risk in all patients who have had their chest opened.

Another factor as mentioned above is fear of pain, which prevents the patient breathing deeply enough, from coughing, or from moving their body at all. Fear and anxiety can be allayed by reasurance, backed up by instructions to hold the chest with their hands or hug a pillow while coughing. The dangers of inadequate breathing can be explained in simple terms of a chest infection that will delay recovery and discharge.

Inhalation therapy is given in the form of steam inhalations or with nebulised intermittent positive pressure breathing, with a Bird or Bennett respirator. The physiotherapist will vigorously treat the patient at least twice a day, usually after analgesia and steam inhalation therapy. The doctor will listen to the patient's chest and take X-rays.

HEART FAILURE

All patients are at risk of developing heart failure after cardiac surgery, especially those in failure prior to the operation. Low cardiac output may be noted by cool, pale peripheries, a lowered urine output, tachycardia and continuing lethargy. The patient may have a troublesome cough, or produce white thin sputum and have an increased respiratory rate. Blood pressure may initially be well maintained, but these patients should be carefully examined by the medical team. Those known to have poor left ventricular function will be mobilized more gently than fitter patients. Digoxin may be commenced to improve cardiac function. Fluid retention and venous congeston can be detected by a lowered urine output, increased thirst and fluid intake, and a weight gain. The jugular venous pressure may be noticeably elevated, and oedema may develop.

Fluids are usually restricted for the first few days: 1500 – 2000 ml in an adult. A fluid balance chart will be recorded during this time but, when the patient is more mobile and allowed free fluids, he will be weighed daily to check for fluid retention. Diuretics with potassium supplements are commonly necessary in the postoperative period, e.g. frusemide 40 mg and amiloride 10 mg are given until the patient returns to preoperative weight, then Navidrex K once daily is given until the patient is reviewed in outpatients. Patients with residual heart failure will require larger doses of diuretics. A chest X-ray should reveal any pulmonary oedema or signs of an enlarged heart shadow. This, together with estimations of urea and electrolytes will be taken until they are all satisfactory.

Table 8.2   Possible complications of the postoperative cardiac patient.

Complication/cause	Signs & symptoms	Treatment
Cardiac failure Poor myocardial function, acidosis, hypoxia, low serum calcium, fluid overload	Vasoconstriction, cool skin temperature, low urine output, low blood pressure, high CVP, tachycardia	Correct cause if possible, diuretics, inotropic agents, dobutamine, dopamine, adrenaline
Tamponade Exessive bleeding, blocked drain	Large blood loss suddenly stops. As for heart failure with high CVP, tachycardia	Unblock drain, open chest to remove clot
Haemorrhage Hypertension, low clotting factors, fibrin, prothrombin, vitamin K, platelets, calcium, circulating heparin from operation, tear or loose suture	As for heart failure but CVP low. Large blood loss to drains	Treat hypertension with sedation or vasodilators. Reverse heparin with protamine sulphate. Cyclokapron 0.5 g i.v.,fresh frozen plasma, platelet concentrate, fresh blood, theatre repair
Cerebrovascular accident Clot from poorly contracted atria or ventricle, vegetations on valve. Hypoxia, hypotension, air embolism	Failure to wake up. Facial or limb weakness. Restlessness, uncooperative. Pupil reaction sluggish or absent if very severe	Dexamethazone i.v. to reduce any cerebral oedema. Nil once occurred. Start passive movements early & physio early. Inform relatives before they visit. *Prevention* by good intraoperative technique

Pulmonary oedema		
Poor left ventricle, fluid overload, renal failure, myocardial infarction	Low cardiac output, central cyanosis, pink frothy sputum, blood gases, chest X-ray, dyspnoea if breathing spontaneously or fighting ventilator. Restless	Diuretics, cardiac stimulants, positive pressure ventilation, IABP
Arrhythmias		
Acidosis, hypoxia, heart failure, inotropic drugs, hypovolaemia, fear, pain, low serum potassium.	Observe monitor, irregular or rapid apex	Treat cause, suppres myocardium with lignocaine, disopyramide & verapamil, over-pace
Heart blocks		
Local oedema, post AVR or septal surgery	Slow heart rate	Pacemaker
Myocardial infarction		
Hypotension, poor coronary blood flow, hypoxia	Heart failure, arrhythmias, ECG changes, slower postoperative progress	Wean from ventilation and inotropic drugs more cautiously than usual. Treat heart failure and arrhythmias. Slower mobilization
Renal failure		
Hypotension, post SB endocarditis, after long bypass deposits of haemolysed cells in kidneys, septicaemia	Low or excessive urine output, pulmonary oedema, high blood urea, serum potassium derangements	Maintain blood pressure and fluid volume. Mannitol, diuretics, Peritoneal dialysis

ARRHYTHMIAS

Abnormal heart rhythms may occur in any patient after surgery. Atrial fibrilation is the commonest disturbance, and occurs in 50% of patients with mitral valve disease.

If the apex rate is recorded for a full minute any irregularities should be evident. The irregularities should be diagnosed and confirmed on a 12 lead ECG.

Occasionally, patients develop heart blocks or tachycardias post surgery. These may seriously affect the cardiac output and produce a state of shock which should be treated as discussed on pp. 125–9.

Patients known to have heart block or bradycardias may be connected to a temporary pacemaker and monitored until the rhythm improves or is treated. Transthoracic pacing wires are usually left in situ for five days, if no disturbance to the rhythm is noted they will be removed by the nurse (*see* p. 89).

An ECG will be recorded on the first postoperative day, after any change in condition or undiagnosed chest pain and before discharge.

THROMBOEMBOLI

Any period of bed rest or reduced mobility can lead to venous stasis and deep vein thrombosis (DVT). Cardiac patients have the added risk of high venous pressures and slow circulation. The wearing of anti-embolic stockings and early mobilization will reduce the incidence of DVT and all patients should be instructed in leg exercises that can be carried out with little expenditure of effort. Immediately post surgery, the nurse should carry out passive exercises two hourly for the patient.

Pulmonary embolism can occur after a venous thrombus. A small embolus could cause some pleuretic pain, a small haemoptysis and secondary chest infection; these would slow the patient's recovery. A larger embolus could endanger life by seriously reducing lung and cardiac function.

Patients in atrial fibrillation and those with prosthetic valves are at risk of thrombi developing. Anticoagulents for lifelong protection will be given to those with prosthetic valves; tissue valves from pigs or humans require anticoagulent cover for a few weeks or months only.

Following coronary artery vein bypass grafting, patients may be anticoagulated or prescribed drugs that inhibit platelet stickiness — so reducing the risk of clot formation, e.g. persantin or aspirin. Warfarin is the anticoagulant most commonly used, and will be commenced on the evening of the second or third postoperative day. This drug prevents the formation of thrombin in the liver, and takes 24 – 36 hours to be effective. Prothrombin time will be tested daily until the patient is stabilized on a suitable dose. Patients with greatly prolonged prothrombin times may haemorrhage. The nurse should look for small amounts of blood that may be detected in the urine, stool, or sputum. Patients with a history of gastric ulceration may require antacids or cimetidine to prevent gastric haemorrhage.

INFECTION

It is usual practice to 'cover' the cardiac surgical patient with prophylactic antibiotics from premedication until 3 – 5 days postoperatively: flucloxacillin and gentamicin are commonly used. A raised temperature, tachycardia and leucocytosis indicate the possible presence of infection, which may gain access to the patient in many ways:

1 During the operation, from dust particles in the theatre or from the nose or throat of personnel directly into the opened chest or heart.

2 From ventilators, humidifiers, or endotracheal suction catheters. Therefore insired gases are filtered, tubings changed daily, and strict aseptic suction techniques employed with vigorous chest physiotherapy to prevent infection and collapse.

3 From i.v. infusions, from the fluid, giving set or three-way taps. The infusion sets are therefore changed every 24 hours and care must be taken not to introduce infection when giving intravenous drugs directly or into infusion bags; life-threatening septicaemia could occur.

4 From wounds, urine catheters, or insertion of intravenous or arterial cannulae. The nurse should be observant for any inflammation, discharge or pain.

The sternal wound is usually closed with self-dissolving sutures, but the drain sites are held together with silk purse string sutures which should be removed 8 – 10 days after surgery. Thoracotomy wounds are under more tension, so will usually be closed with silk sutures, and removed on the 10th day. Chest wounds are dressed on the first day, cleaned and covered with a sterile pre-packed dry dressing. The next day the wound is usually clean and dry and can be fully exposed on the third day.

The leg wounds resulting from vein extraction for coronary artery bypass grafting can also be treated this way, but the patient should wear anti-embolic stockings and have their legs elevated when sitting down.

Any pyrexia should be reported and swabs taken of any suspicious site. The tips of catheters or venous lines will be sent for bacteriological assessment and blood cultures should be taken if high temperatures or rigors occur and the patient suddenly deteriorates.

ANOREXIA

A paralytic ileus can occur postoperatively, so check that bowel sound are present before fluids or diet are commenced. These are checked in the ICU before the patient goes to the ward, but should be re-checked if the patient is anorexic or distended.

A full and balanced diet is essential to build and repair tissues and blood cells. At first the patient will be reluctant to eat, but should be encouraged with appetisers or favourite foods brought from home, to include an ample amount of fresh fruit. To increase appetite the patient should be sat out in a chair for his meals from the second postoperative day and, if he is progressing well, he should be encouraged to eat at a ward table with other patients. Ale or stout may be offered before meals.

Constipation may be troublesome following the immobility of the operation and the use of narcotic and codeine-based analgesics. Dorbanex from the second postoperative night appears to suit most patients. If a complication prevents the patient becoming mobile, diet and aperients will need more careful attention in consultation with the medical staff and the dietician.

Renal impairment can occur. A low protein, high calorie diet may be ordered but the patient may need assistance to adhere to this.

TIREDNESS AND DEPRESSION

The patient should be warned before the operation that he will feel tired, lethargic, and even depressed a few days afterwards. One of the main reasons is that the body has been through a tremendous upheaval so it is not surprising that it requires rest. However, although patients can accept feeling unwell immediately postoperatively, they are often overwhelmed by their inability to be enthusiastic towards their family or friends. They feel ashamed of their feelings, and may weep openly. This experience may be entirely new to some, especially men, who will need understanding and reassurance from the nurses that these feelings and reactions, though real and frightening, are not uncommon and will pass in a few days. On return to the ward from the ICU the patient may feel anxious about the loss of a one to one nurse: patient ratio, and the removal of all the monitoring devices. The ward nurses should reassure the patient by remaining in view, giving the patient a nurse-call bell, and informing the patient that all is well after every observation of pulse or blood pressure. The senior nurse on duty and the doctor should see the patient to discuss his progress at least once a shift. As the recovery progresses, these discussions need only be brief — the patient's own feeling of well being and return of confidence will reassure him with only a little reinforcement from the staff.

Continued lethargy could be a sign of low cardiac output or anaemia. The ward routine and visiting should allow the patients long periods of uninterrupted rest during the day as well as at night. Visitors should be advised to stay for short periods only, and not to be concerned if the patient appears tired, depressed, or irritable with them. The nurse must remember that the relatives too have also been through a most anxious and trying time. This may cause them to seek repeated explanations and reassurances, which should readily be given by the nursing and medical staff. A full discussion with the patient and relatives by a senior nurse and the doctor will be necessary before discharge.

MOBILIZATION

The goal of an uneventful postoperative recovery is for the patient to be fully mobile and caring for himself independently within 7 or 8 days. To achieve this the patient must be encouraged to move himself about the bed from the first day. On the second day he will be assisted out of the bed to sit in a chair for meals. The physiotherapist will aid the patient to walk initially, because excessive stooping to protect the sternal wound may occur unless the patient is taught to stand straight. Deep breathing can be carried out while the patient walks slowly round the ward. From the third postoperative day onwards, the patient will be walking to the toilet, assisted with a big bath, and spending most of the day out of bed, except for rest periods, The physiotherapist will assist the patient to walk up and down a flight of stairs, to regain balance and self-confidence.

DISCHARGE

Depending on the patient's overall conditon, he may be ready for discharge 8 – 12 days after the operation. Some patients require convalescence in a special hospital; this will depend upon how ill the patient was pre- and postoperatively, but a more important consideration is what are the home circumstances. If the patient lives on his own in a fifth floor flat without a lift and has no relatives to stay with him, then he will require a place in a convalescent hospital for about two weeks. If the patient has a spouse or relative who can plan time off work to assist and offer moral support, then home is the most suitable place to go.

Any drugs the patient is being discharged with should be fully explained to the patient. He should know when to take them, and where to obtain new supplies.

Occasionally patients are discharged before their sutures are removed and arrangements for the district nurse to visit will therefore have to be made.

The amount of physical activity the patient should be encouraged to take will depend on his age and preoperative fitness. A person who has had a long illness, e.g. bacterial endocarditis and then valve replacement, will require at least three months to regain their energy and vigour. Long periods of rest during the day should punctuate periods of activity such as gentle walks, that can be extended as the patient recovers. A fitter person who was not in heart failure prior to an operation such as a coronary artery bypass graft, should be encouraged to walk long distances each day, assist with household chores, but still have a rest period during the day for the first month. Sexual activity can be re-started as soon as the patient wishes, without any risk.

A date for return to work can be discussed prior to discharge, then fully at outpatients, but 6 – 8 weeks after discharge should be aimed at. Lighter work or shorter hours may be necessary for some, but a full return, where possible, should be encouraged.

An outpatient appointment is arranged for six weeks' time and a letter is sent to the General Practitioner. The patient should seek advice from his own doctor if he is at all worried, so an earlier appointment or re-admission can be arranged if necessary.

HEART TRANSPLANT SURGERY

The majority of patients with heart disease respond to medical or surgical therapy, but the heart muscle in some patients is so badly damaged that the only hope of any type of survival is for the heart muscle itself to be replaced.

Heart transplants were first attempted in 1967 by Dr Christian Barnaard in South Africa, but the first patient lived only 18 hours. Since then over 500 operations have been carried out, mostly in America, where the first year survival record is about 67% and the four-year survival rate is 56%. The longest living recipient in the world received his heart over 14 years ago.

In Britain, Mr. Donald Ross carried out three heart transplants in the early 1970s, but unfortunately the patient survival times were unacceptably short. Further series of heart transplants were started in Britain in 1979 at both Papworth Hospital in Cambridge and Harefield

Hospital in West London, after advances in immunosuppressive therapy and organ transport had been made in America.

SELECTION

At present, only patients who are under 50 years old and otherwise healthy will be selected for transplant surgery since osteoporosis and adverse effects of immunosuppression are more likely to occur in patients over this age. About 70% of patients referred to transplant teams are turned down because of disease in another body system, discovered in the extensive preoperative screening. Insulin-dependent diabetics are not currently accepted.

Longstanding heart disease frequently causes secondary changes in the lungs. These changes are especially common in congenital heart disease so a heart transplant would not help many of these patients; however heart/lung transplants are being cautiously tried in America.

Patients selected for surgery may already have undergone standard operations for coronary artery bypass grafting at least once, and many will have suffered myocardial infarctions that have damaged the pumping efficiency of the myocardium beyond the stage where further revascularization can help.

Cardiomyopathy is a group of diseases that cause the heart muscle to pump ineffectively. Medical therapy will usually initially keep heart failure in check but ultimately a transplant for some is the only chance of survival.

Preoperative preparation

Other specialists such as nephrologists, neurologists, ENT surgeons, and endocrinologists will be consulted if there is any suspicion or history of other disease. If the coronary arteries have been diseased by atheroma or the heart damaged by smoking or hypertension, then it is likely that other organs will be affected.

All patients will undergo respiratory function testing, dental assessment, and swab culture from every potentially infected site. Blood samples will be taken for tissue typing as well as the usual preoperative screening.

The patient will be seen by a psychiatrist for he and his family must have a sincere desire to live and must all be able to withstand the mental strain of waiting, the possible complications, and the statistically relatively high risk of death. In addition, even if all goes well, for several days or weeks following the transplant, the patient will be in isolation and even the spouse will need to wear overshoes, cap, mask, gown and gloves before touching the patient. This isolation can cause tremendous strain. The psychiatrist's report forms a good basis from which to judge behaviour pattern changes that may occur postoperatively — from the isolation and the possible effects of steroid therapy.

The social worker will need to become involved with the patient and the family. Usually the illness leading up to the transplant will have been prolonged, mostly attacking men who are otherwise in the prime of life and at the peak of their social responsibilities, career, and earning capacity. The family will probably have been making sacrifices, both financial and social, to protect and care for the patient. The social worker therefore is not only a means of helping the family to obtain monetary and housing benefits, but can give moral support and advice on family matters.

All the patients are, of course, aware that, for them to receive a heart, someone else must die. This can frequently provoke feelings of guilt. Some patients wish to know the details of the donor, but many do not. These feelings should be openly discussed prior to the transplant, perhaps at the same time as the effects of isolation and steroid therapy are explained.

The next of kin should be clearly identified. As with other major surgery, the family or friend will need to be prepared to shoulder the worries and fears, and support the patient. The nurse plays a large part not only in the testing and recording of physical signs such as blood pressure, urinalysis or observing for signs of infection or disease, but also in acting as part of a well informed team when information and advice is asked for by patients and families, as well as providing psychological support and company.

Cardiac screening will largely have been undertaken by the referring hospital. The history and results of exercise tolerance, angiography, cardiac output studies, thalium scanning, echocardiography, and computerized axial tomography, will be reviewed and repeated if necessary during a three-day assessment period. If the patient is then accepted to the transplant programme he will be allowed to go home if possible, but many patients are too ill to leave hospital and may die in hospital before a suitable donor heart is available.

THE DONOR HEART

Hearts usually become available from otherwise healthy individuals (under 40 years old) who have suffered brain damage leading to brain death, commonly as a result of road traffic accidents. These patients will already be on ventilators, as spontaneous respiration will have ceased. Brain death will be established by two senior doctors who are not involved in the transplant programme in any way, and who will separately carry out a series of tests to be absolutely certain that brain stem death has occurred and that recovery is impossible. The family will then be told that their relative is effectively dead for, although the heart and other organs are functioning normally, the brain is dead. This has already resulted in loss of control of respiration, soon cardiovascular regulation will also cease to function normally, and then the heart will stop after a period of hours or days. Many people are aware of the possibility of organ transplants, and the relatives sometimes offer the organs for this purpose before the doctor asks them for their consent.

If the heart is considered suitable, i.e. there have been no periods of hypoxia, prolonged hypotension, or cardiac arrest, and there is a previous clear relevant medical history as far as can be ascertained, then the donor's blood will be sent to be cross-matched and tissue typed with a prospective recipient's blood. Europe has a computerized data bank with tissue type details of would-be recipients, so that the best match possible can be made of the small supply of suitable donor organs.

The heart transplant team remove the heart from the donor by, firstly, clamping the venae cavae, so allowing the heart to empty, then the aorta is clamped and the vessels severed. The pulmonary veins at the back of the heart are cut and the heart removed. The aorta and coronary arteries are perfused with ice cold Hartmann's solution with added potassium which cools and preserves the heart by stopping both electrical and mechanical activity. The heart is then wrapped in sterile bags and transported in under four hours in ice to the waiting recipient.

Research into the transport and storage of donor hearts allowing a greater time lapse between removal and the replacement is advancing rapidly, and will greatly help the transplant programme and donor organ availability.

PREPARATION OF THE RECIPIENT

As soon as a donor is available the recipient and family will be informed and prepared. This preparation is essentially similar to that for any open heart surgery, although additional precautions such as using autoclaved linen and a theatre cap are taken when the transplant is confirmed.

Before the premedication is given, a mild oral analgesic and a nystatin lozenge are given. An i.v. line is aseptically established and a loading dose of the immunosuppressive agent antithymocite globulin (either from the horse (HATG) or from the rabbit (RATG)) and the opiate premedication are given. The dose of HATG or RATG is usually 100 mg i.v. and 200 mg i.m. An anaphylactic reaction could occur so the nurse must stay with the patient and have Piriton, hydrocortisone and adrenaline to hand.

THE OPERATION

Anaesthesia is induced as usual but the anaesthetist will wear gloves and mask and take extra care not to introduce infection while intubating or inserting venous and arterial lines.

Cardiopulmonary bypass will be established in the normal manner with blood taken from the tied venae cavae and returned via a pump and oxygenator to the aorta above the aortic cross-clamp. The preparation of the recipient patient takes place at the same time as the donor heart is being removed, so that the recipient is ready for immediate insertion of the donor heart when the team returns.

The recipient heart is prepared by retaining the venae cavae and posterior portion of both atria, including the pulmonary veins. The sinus node, atrioventricular valves and ventricles are discarded. All autonomic nervous control to the heart is removed.

The aorta and pulmonary arteries are divided and shaped to fit the donor heart, and the donor heart trimmed to fit the remaining portions of the recipient heart. A continuous line of suturing is started from the left atrium.

The patient will now be warmed and weaned from cardiopulmonary bypass in the normal manner. The rhythm and contractile force of the heart are checked, and the suture lines are examined for leaks.

REJECTION AND INFECTION

There are two potential life-threatening complications of transplantation in addition to those of normal cardiac surgery: rejection of the new heart and overwhelming infection.

Careful tissue typing will ensure that the donor's tissues match those of the recipient as closely as possible; however, the recipient's defence mechanisms will still recognize the new heart as foreign tissue. White cells will develop antibodies to destroy and reject the new heart unless the immune system is suppressed. Immunosuppression is achieved by reducing the patient's white cells with ATG from the horse, rabbit, or goat. After the loading dose with the premedication, 100 mg is given daily for two weeks and, if there are signs of rejection, the drug is continued for 3 – 5 days more. Imuran will also be given and the blood levels checked. Prednisone is administered in large doses and it should be possible to reduce this to 10 mg per day by the end of a year. Imuran and prednisone doses alter daily initially according to the T cell white count.

Rejection can occur at any time, even immediately on return from theatre. The nurse should suspect rejection if the voltage of the QRS complex becomes reduced, the patient's cardiovascular signs alter, or his general feeling of wellbeing changes. Myocardial biopsy will confirm that rejection is occurring. Large doses of methylprednisolone will be given to halt the rejection and further ATG will be prescribed.

Because the patient is immunosuppressed he is vulnerable to any *infection*. For this reason he is carefully washed and prepared preoperatively and isolated afterwards with strict and meticulous reverse barrier nursing. Any person who suspects they have even a minor infection, e.g. a sore throat or herpes sore, should not attend these transplant patients. Any infection can endanger the patient or delay progress. Prophylactic antibiotics and an antifungal agent such as Acyclovir are given; daily swabs and samples are cultured, and additional antibiotics given if appropriate. Infection and inflammation will of course be masked by the steroids.

Following surgery the patient is received into an air-conditioned isolation room that has been especially cleaned and stocked. The room will contain an air lock and an area for scrubbing up and gowning; it will hold spare stocks and will have direct access to the grounds. It takes approximately three hours for the nurse to shower and gown herself, then clean and prepare the room. The patient will stay there for 10 – 14 days so *all* the equipment the patient will require in the acute and recovery stages should be present and sterilized.

Apart from these strict barrier nursing procedures, the immediate postoperative care of the patient is the same as for other cardiac surgery cases. However, the patient now has a strong heart and will warm and wake quickly; endotracheal extubation may be considered after only a few hours. Removal of drains and other lines will follow as soon as possible to minimize infection risk.

POSTOPERATIVE RECOVERY

Within 12 hours the patient should be wide awake and ready to be helped out of bed to walk round the room. The postoperative plan will have been discussed in detail, as will the physiotherapy, exercise, diet and drug regimes. Patients frequently quickly develop great appetites and energy reserves postoperatively.

Exercise begins as soon as the patient's medical state permits. A walk round the room 24 hours after exubation is increased to a mile on the exercise bike on the third postoperative day. Arm and leg exercises as well as the usual breathing exercises are supervised by a physiotherapist. Without interrupting reverse barrier nursing (i.e. the patient wears a mask and gown), the patient will be encouraged to walk around the hospital grounds within the first postoperative week, quickly building up to more vigorous exercise. The patient may experience skeletal muscle pains because many muscles will have been virtually unused during the long illness prior to transplantation.

Unfortunately, skeletal pain sometimes occurs due to osteoporosis following the large doses of steroids, despite the patient being given calcium supplements. This osteoporosis is reversible to a certain degree when the dose of steroids is reduced.

DIET

The patient will be encouraged to eat from the first postoperative day. A low fat, low cholesterol diet will be individually prepared and sealed by the hospital kitchens. Fresh foods are not allowed initially as they might harbour infection. The patient's spouse will be encouraged to serve the patient with tablets and drinks as well as heating and serving meals and generally preparing for home. Crockery and cutlery will be sterilized by autoclaving or soaking in sodium hypochlorite solution.

PROGRESS

After 10 – 14 days, the immunosuppressive therapy should hopefully be stabilized and the patient's white cell count rising without a pyrexia or other signs of infection. When this occurs, the patient is less vulnerable to infection and can be released from the strict barrier nursing, though masks are still worn. The patient may wear outdoor clothes and only a mask when cycling or exercising in the grounds.

After a short period of the relaxed barrier nursing, it is hoped the patient should be fit with no signs of infection or rejection and be happy and ready for discharge. Thereafter, he will have many tablets to take and must have physical examinations and blood tests regularly. These are performed at his local hospital, in close communication with the transplant team.

A myocardial biopsy, under strict sterile conditions in the operating theatre or angiography department, is performed postoperatively at monthly intervals during the first year, and whenever there is a suspicion of rejection.

The patient is re-admitted annually for 48 hours for a full check-up, including angiography and myocardial biopsy. Coronary artery disease can re-occur but, because the heart is denervated, the patient will not experience angina. Cardiomyopathy does not recur.

The patient and family have been given continual advice on exercise, diet, and how to avoid infection or further illness, they have also been involved in their own care during the later stages of inpatient stay. Any infection or slight sign of rejection may necessitate re-admission to hospital, but after about four months the patient should be contemplating return to work. It is vital for the patient to realize the full importance of reporting any infection or feeling of any degree of malaise, however minor, and of continuing medication.

My thanks to the staff at Harefield Hospital for their willing help with this section, especially Mr Yacoub and Miss M.M. Jones.

Index

233